# Renal Diet Cookbook for Beginners

*Complete Guide with 2000 Days of delicious, Low Sodium, Potassium, and Phosphorous recipes to start Kidney-Friendly Lifestyle*

By

Patricia Harper

# Table Of Contents

# INTRODUCTION

The human body's health hangs in the balance when all its interconnected biological functions work in perfect harmony. Without the regular function of its key organs, the body quickly sustains irreparable harm. Kidney dysfunction is one such example, and not only does it disrupt the overall water balance, but a variety of other disorders also develop as a result of this issue. Kidney problems are progressive, which implies that if they are not treated and managed, they might lead to kidney damage before their time. It is crucial to control and manage the problem and restrict its progression, which can be achieved via medicinal and natural means. A change in lifestyle and diet is essential.

A kidney-friendly diet and lifestyle keep excess minerals out of the kidneys and improve medications' effectiveness. Consequently, treatment in the absence of a healthy diet is useless.

Your intake of protein, sodium, potassium, and phosphorus are all regulated by a good renal diet. It's not about eating specialty foods; instead, making sensible improvements to your everyday meals, including whole grains, fresh fruits, and veggies. The renal diet helps control bowel movements and improve other essential body functions.

Following Renal diet may limit the waste your body produces, minimizing the strain on your kidneys and retaining renal function. The renal diet may help delay complete renal failure or dialysis by several years and prevent the condition from progressing to the next stage.

Thinking about what to eat while following a low-protein, low-sodium, low-potassium, and low-phosphorus diet may be overwhelming. Making one minor adjustment or cutting out a few food types from your diet won't suffice.

This book overcomes the uncertainty and tension associated with selecting recipes and menu items while dining out. It will most significantly support your long-term success in keeping up with nutritional modifications. You are not forced to live on boring food for years if you follow a limiting renal diet that is both tasty and unique. It's crucial to empower oneself with information about renal nutrition. This book is accessible to anyone, regardless of their cooking experience or educational level.

Before starting a new diet or making changes to an existing one, always consult with your doctor.

# CHAPTER 1
# Understanding Renal Disease

Kidneys keep you healthy by filtering up to 47.56 gallons of blood daily, excreting extra fluid and waste. It produces urine that holds the by-products of the body's metabolism (water, chemicals, and salt) in the blood. Many healthy individuals are unaware that their kidneys do not function effectively, leading to kidney failure, which lowers filtration quality.

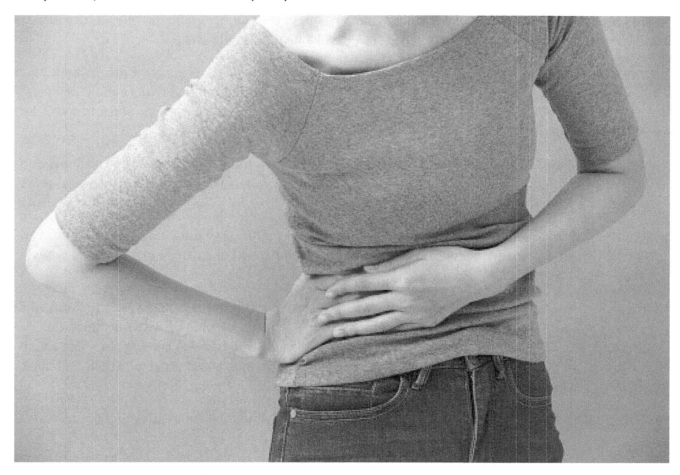

Kidney disease remains one of the leading causes of mortality in the united states. The likelihood rises with age. A great deal of damage may be done if it remains unaddressed. The sooner you start caring for your kidney, the better you will manage it successfully. The organ kidney looks like the shape of a bean and is two in number, each about a fist's size. They are positioned slightly behind the rib cage, on each side of the spine.

## 1.1 Know About Your Kidney

The kidneys eliminate excess fluid and waste from the body via urine. Urine production includes complex discharge and reabsorption. These procedures are crucial for body chemical stability. The kidneys remove acid from the body's cells and maintain a healthy blood salt, water, and mineral balance. Kidney hormone affects other organs. It regulates calcium metabolism, controls blood pressure, improves red blood cell growth, and strengthens bones.

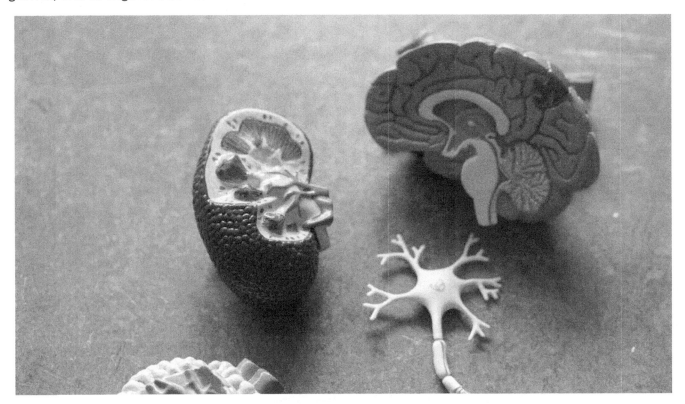

Each kidney nephron contains a "glomerulus" The glomerulus filters the blood, while the tubule feeds nutrients and removes waste. The glomerulus empties blood into the tubule. A healthy kidney pumps and eliminates half a cup of blood per minute; the urine is carried to the bladder through the ureters.

## 1.2 Chronic Kidney Disease Disorder.

The kidneys gradually become less effective over time, leading to chronic renal disease (CKD) disorder. CKD lowers the kidneys' ability to maintain health since they can no longer work effectively. If kidney disease worsens, the levels of waste and excess fluid in the blood will increase, making you sick. As the kidney damage worsens, many consequences might develop, including nerve damage, poor digestion, weak bones, low blood count (anemia), and high blood pressure. Other risks, such as an elevated risk of cardiovascular and blood vessel disease, can develop gradually over time. Early diagnosis and treatment of progressive kidney disease might delay the onset of organ failure, the requirement for dialysis, or the need for a kidney transplant to maintain life. More than 30 million individuals in America have been diagnosed with significant kidney diseases, and millions are at increased risk. Kidney disease is more common among older persons, those from the Pacific Islands, Americans, Indians, African Americans, and Hispanics, as well as those with diabetes, high blood pressure, and a family history of kidney failure.

## Causes of Renal Disease

When protein in the urine (proteinuria) lasts for an extended period, you may have a chronic kidney disorder. Elevated blood pressure and diabetes are the main two risk factors for developing chronic kidney disease, accounting for around 75% of cases.

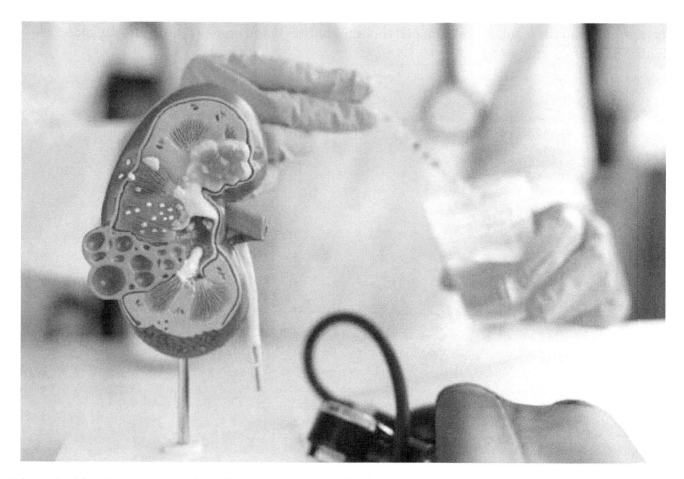

When the blood pressure against the blood vessel walls rises, hypertension, also known as high blood pressure, occurs. If left untreated and uncontrolled, hypertension may lead to chronic renal failure, strokes, and cardiac problems. High blood sugar levels resulting from diabetes damage the heart, kidneys, eyes, nerves, and blood vessels. Chronic renal disease may cause hypertension, and the condition can cause hypertension. Immune inflammation is disrupted by the kidneys' filtration mechanism in disorder known as glomerulonephritis, which arises from immune system failure. The disease will only impact the kidneys and extend throughout the body (lupus nephritis, vacuities). Glomerulonephritis and high blood pressure often coexist.

## Symptoms of Renal Disease

Compared to the advanced stages of the condition, symptoms are often invisible and mild in the early stages of kidney disease. You can, however, observe some of the following symptoms:

- Increased Urination, particularly at night,
- Dry and Itchy Skin
- Muscle cramps, mostly during the night
- Swollen feet and ankles
- Lack of appetite
- Puffiness around the eyes, especially in the morning
- Lacking concentration
- Insomnia
- General weakness and lack of energy

Chronic kidney disease, regardless of age, can occur to anybody. However, some are more vulnerable to the illness than others.

## Stages and diagnosis

The ultimate damage, which contributes to kidney failure, does not arise instantly. For an extended period, it is slow and progressive. Suppose early diagnosis of chronic kidney disease happens. In that case, significant improvements in daily life and medications will maintain you at your health for a long time.

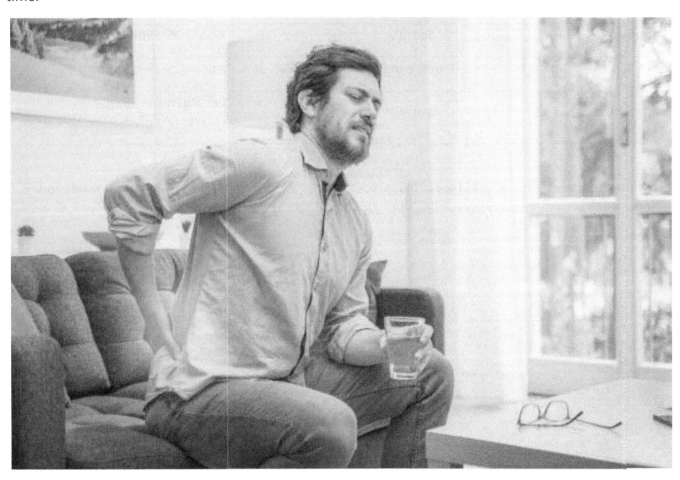

There are 5 CKD stages, and each level is handled and taken care of differently. Glomerular filtration rate (GFR) determines the kidney failure stage and the kidney's level of function. It is a mathematical formula for determining a glomerular filtration rate by serum creatinine, gender, race, age, and other individual factors. A doctor takes a blood sample and tests to determine the amount of serum creatinine. GFR lets your doctor assess the extent of your kidney's disease and function and suggests the appropriate diagnosis and treatment. Creatinine is removed from the blood while the kidneys are in good health. In other words, when renal activity slows, the blood's creatinine increases.

*Five Stages of Chronic Kidney Disease*

| Stage | Description | Glomerular filtration rate (GFR) |
|---|---|---|
| Normal Kidney Function | Healthy Kidneys | About 90mL/min or more. |
| Stage 1 | normal/high GFR with Kidney Damage | About 90mL/min or more. |
| Stage 2 | mild decrease in the GFR | About 60-89mL/min. |
| Stage 3 | Moderate decrease in the GFR | About 30-59mL/min. |
| Stage 4 | Severe decrease in the GFR | About 15-29mL/min. |
| Stage 5 | Kidney Failure | Less than the 15mL/min receiving dialysis. |

Depending on the stage of your kidney disease, your doctor will decide how to treat you. Consult your doctor if you have any concerns regarding your kidney disease stage or treatment.

# CHAPTER 2
## Renal Diet

A proper diet is a secret to good health while particularly necessary for a chronic kidney disorder. Your body lacks its original functionality when you have kidney disease. However, kidneys could be protected by adjusting diet. People with impaired kidney function must follow a renal or kidney diet to reduce the quantity of waste in their blood. Wastes from consumed meals and drinks end up in the blood. The kidneys do not filter or eliminate waste when impaired renal function. The patient's electrolyte balances may suffer when waste is left in the blood.

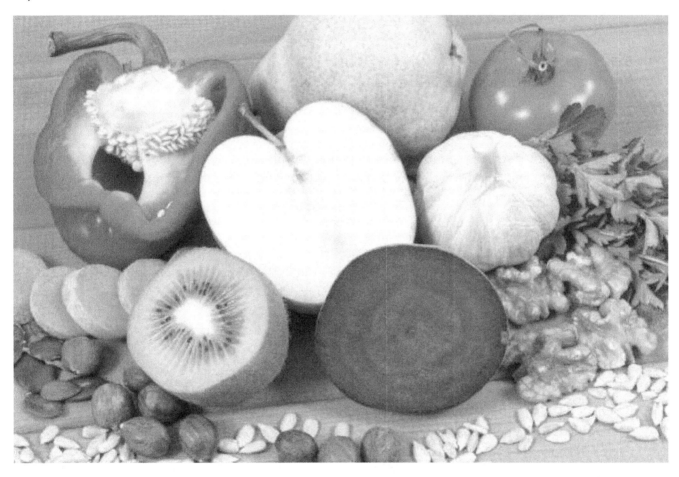

A renal-friendly diet supports kidney health and delays kidney failure's onset. Staying safe for as long as it can be achieved by having the necessary lifestyle that makes you give up on so many favorite foods.

A renal diet is low in protein, phosphorus, and sodium. A renal diet also emphasizes obtaining high-quality protein and often restricting fluid intake. Limiting potassium and calcium may also be necessary for certain people. However, it depends on the patient's condition specifically. Because every person's body is different, every patient must collaborate with a renal health professional to design a diet suited to their requirements. The outcome of the test on an individual with kidney disease will decide, as defined by their doctor, the type of specific diet needed at each chronic renal disease level.

The following substances are vital to keeping an eye on to support a renal diet:

## 2.1- General Diet Guidelines

Following the dietitian or doctor's instructions is necessary, especially if a specific diet has been assigned. The following are general food terms if you have been hospitalized with kidney disease.

### Sodium

One of the body's three primary electrolytes is sodium (potassium and chloride are the other two). Electrolytes control the flow of fluids into and out of the body's tissues and cells. The mineral sodium may be present in certain organic foods. The majority of individuals relate sodium with salt. But salt is a combination of sodium and chloride. Salt and other forms of sodium may be present in your food. Additionally, processed meals have higher salt content.

Sodium helps with:

- Balancing body fluids quantity
- Regulates blood volume and blood pressure.
- Regulates muscle contraction and nerve function.
- Regulates acid-base blood balance.

For patients with kidney disease, too much salt can be dangerous since their kidneys cannot properly eliminate extra sodium and fluid from the body. As a result of which, sodium and fluid buildup in the bloodstream and tissues, and they can cause:

- High blood pressure
- swelling in the face, legs, and hands: Edema
- Heart failure: The heart will overwork with extra fluid in the bloodstream, rendering it weak and enlarged.
- Increased thirst
- Breath Shortness: fluid in the lungs will build up, causing it hard to breathe.

### Monitor sodium intake:

- Read Food Descriptions: It always mentions the sodium content.
- Be careful about serving sizes.
- Go for fresh meat instead of a packed one.
- Avoid refined foods.
- Choose vegetables and fresh fruit or canned and frozen products with no salt added.
- Use brand product items that are low in sodium.
- Do **NOT** add salt to foods that are cooked at home.
- Use spices that do not have "salt" in their description (instead of garlic salt, choose garlic powder.)
- Limit the average amount of sodium to 150 mg per snack and 400 mg per meal.

### Potassium

Potassium is a vital component naturally found in the body and is present in everything you eat. Keeps the heartbeat regular and ensures that muscles are working properly. Potassium is necessary to maintain fluid and electrolyte balance in the bloodstream. Your kidneys help maintain the ideal potassium level in your body and eliminate excess amounts via urination.

## Monitor potassium intake.

Unnecessary potassium will not be removed because of kidney failure, so potassium level rises in the body. High blood potassium is recognized as hyperkalemia, which may trigger:

- Slow pulse
- Muscle weakness
- Heart attacks
- An irregular heartbeat
- Death

A patient must control the potassium amount that enters the body when the kidneys no longer balance potassium.

## Tips to keep balanced potassium levels in your blood:

Make a meal schedule with the help of a renal dietitian.

- Restrict foods rich in potassium.
- Limit dairy goods or milk up to 8 oz a day.
- Use fruits and vegetables that are fresh.
- Limit salt substitutes & potassium seasonings.
- Read labeling & avoid processed foods that contain potassium chloride.
- Keep a diet journal.
- Be careful about serving size.

## Phosphorus

A mineral called phosphorus is essential for the growth and development of bones. Additionally, it helps in the growth of connective tissue, organ development, and muscular action. Following consumption and digestion of phosphorus-containing food, phosphorus is absorbed by the small intestine and deposited in the bones.

## Monitor Phosphorus intake

When working normally, it is normal for kidneys to eliminate too much phosphorus from the blood. When kidney function is impaired, the kidneys cannot excrete excess phosphorus. High phosphorus levels may weaken your bones by removing calcium from them, which causes dangerous calcium concentrations in the heart, lungs, blood vessels, skin, and blood. Phosphorus is present in many foods. Therefore, individuals with compromised renal function should consult a renal dietitian to limit phosphorus intake properly.

## Tips for retaining phosphorus at healthy levels:

- Know which foods have less phosphorus.

- Be careful about the size of servings.
- Take fewer portions of food for meals and snacks rich in protein.
- Consume fresh vegetables and fruits.
- Ask your physician at mealtime to use phosphate binders.
- Avoid processed foods with additional phosphorus. On ingredient labels, check for phosphorus or terms with "PHOS."

## Protein

Protein doesn't cause any problems for healthy kidneys. When protein is absorbed, waste products are produced and purified by the kidney nephrons. With the aid of extra renal proteins, the waste turns into urine. Protein waste builds up in the blood when the kidneys are impaired because they cannot filter it out.

The quantity of protein required for people with Chronic Kidney Disorder varies depending on their disease stage. While protein is required to maintain tissues and other body functions, a nephrologist or renal dietitian stresses the need to consume the recommended quantity for the patient's stage of the disease.

## Fluids

Fluid management is necessary for people with advanced chronic kidney disease since frequent fluid consumption may lead to potentially dangerous fluid accumulation in the body. Dialysis patients also have decreased urine output; thus, adding more fluid to their bodies can put needless strain on their hearts and lungs.

Patients' fluid intake is calculated based on their urine output and dialysis circumstances. Follow the recommendations of your nephrologist and nutritionist for the recommended fluid consumption.

To control the consumption of fluids, patients should:

- Do not drink more than the doctor advises.
- List all foods melting at room temperature.
- Be aware of the volume of fluids used in cooking.

## Recommended dietary intake

| Nutrients | Recommended Intake |
|-----------|--------------------|
| Energy | ≥35 kg/kcal/day; A lesser dose could be suggested if the patient is older than 60 or their body weight is higher than 120 % of what is considered normal. |
| Protein | 1.2 g/kg/day for  clinically stable patients |
| Fat | 25-30% of the total energy intake |

| Carbohydrate | Calorie balance from non-protein sources |
|---|---|
| Total fiber | 20 to 25 g/day |
| Sodium | 750-2000 mg/day |
| Potassium | 2000-2750 mg/day |
| Phosphorus | 800-1000 mg/day |
| Calcium | < 1000 mg/day |
| Water | 750-1500 mL/day |

## 2.2-Foods to Avoid or Cut Down

The items listed below should be avoided or used moderately if you are on a renal diet.

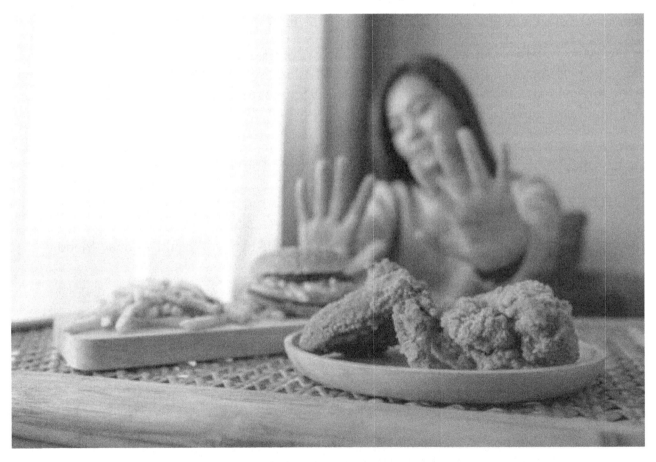

**Dairy**: When on a renal diet, it is often suggested to reduce your dairy consumption; this can help regulate your protein intake and manage the amount of fat you consume. Instead of cottage cheese or brie, consider full-fat cheddar and Parmesan.

**Caffeine**: Caffeine is a stimulant and is challenging to filter by the kidneys. In comparison, caffeine intake on an empty stomach is correlated with the development of kidney stones, and it may also contribute to a rise in calcium content in the urine. Try to steadily decrease the volume of caffeine you drink, allowing the kidneys' better functioning for longer. Green tea is a perfect substitute for coffee, and tea without caffeine is best; it improves stamina like caffeine would help you feel great.

**Avocado:** Avocados are known for their other nutritional advantages in addition to their heart-healthy fiber, fats, and antioxidant content. Although avocados are often a healthy addition to a diet, those with renal disorders must avoid them. Avocados are a rich source of potassium due to their high potassium content. They have an astounding 727 milligrams of potassium per cup (150 g). That is double the potassium that a medium-sized banana has. A cup of avocados has 37% of the 2000 mg potassium limit. Guacamole and avocados should also be avoided while on a renal diet, especially if your doctor has instructed you to reduce your potassium consumption.

**Artificial Sweetener**: If you need anything to sweeten your teas or meals, skip artificial sweeteners like saccharin and go for Stevia.

**Soda:** Soda is toxic to both your kidneys and your bones. Your chance of chronic kidney disease is believed to raise dramatically with soda daily. In a kidney-friendly diet, stop consuming soda.

**GMOs**: Genetically modified organisms are expected to raise the number of free radicals in various foods; kidneys cannot efficiently filter the contaminants and pollutants in these foods.

**Potatoes:** White potatoes and sweet potatoes are rich in potassium. Soaking them in warm water or boiling them twice before frying will remove excess potassium. Sweet potatoes provide many other vitamins and minerals. Still, it is important to contact a doctor or dietitian to determine whether and what levels of potatoes should be used in your diet.

**Tomatoes:** Tomatoes also have a strong potassium content. Canned tomatoes with no salt or sugar can be eaten in moderation. Contact your doctor or dietician to find out if you should stop tomatoes.

## 2.3-Consider Your Lifestyle

Follow the instructions to make the change as simple as possible to have a healthy kidney-friendly lifestyle:

- Eat a heavy breakfast, a small dinner, and a medium-sized lunch.
- Increase vegetable and fruit intake regularly.
- Go for food dressings based on olive oil.
- Instead of fast and processed snacks such as roasted kale chips, and simple yogurt, consider fruits and nuts in moderation, as they are healthier snacks.
- Those needing to regulate calorie consumption and those who have lost their appetite consume smaller meals and light snacks.
- Avoid beverages and sodas since they contain high sugar levels and refined ingredients.
- Drink fresh water and green teas but be careful about how much liquid you can drink daily.
- Do not eat after 8 pm to give your body and kidneys time to work till you sleep.
- Get into the practice of reviewing food labels and checking for salt, potassium, phosphorous, protein, and calorie concentrations.
- Depending on your diagnosis and personal preferences, get a regular diet that contains protein, good fats, and carbohydrates.
- Avoiding smoking.

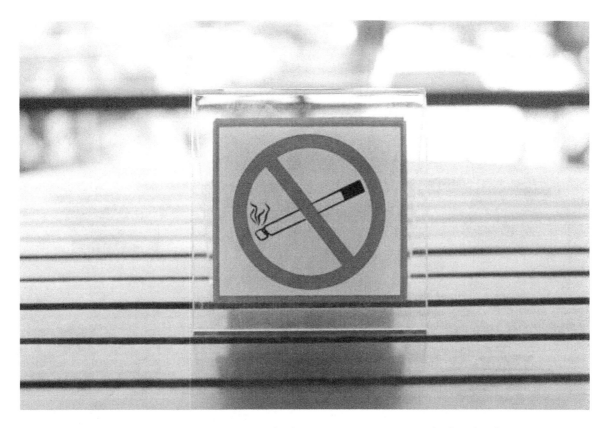

- In a notebook, record the symptoms and what you consume regularly. This lets you maintain track of how many and what sorts of things you have consumed and how they make you feel.
- To ensure it is not too high, keep up with regular appointments and monitor the blood pressure.
- If you have diabetes, ensure you control your health and speak with your doctor on precise sugar guidelines.
- The activity level you can safely accomplish with chronic kidney disease depends on your diagnosis, comorbidities, and general health. Exercising in the initial stages of the disease may assist overcome fatigue's first symptoms.

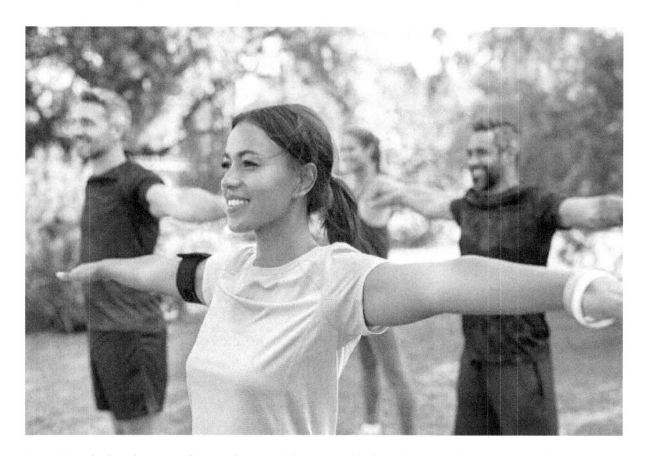

Exercising helps those seeking to lose weight to avoid chronic renal disease-related issues. Exercise improves the heart and reduces stress and anxiety. People who limit their fluid intake shouldn't engage in strenuous activities since they will get dehydrated. Yoga and mild walks are recommended to be active and healthy without overexerting. Seek medical advice.

# CHAPTER 3

# Renal Meal Plan

Controlling your diet and drinking habits is essential if you have a chronic kidney disorder. The kidney-friendly 28-day meal plan and recipes for 2000 days support you while you make dietary adjustments. The meal plan includes the recipes, so you can continue eating well daily. With these meal plans, you can stay on schedule, save money, prepare fast, save time, and decrease waste.

## Preparing for the Diet

Avoid tired, poor practices to enjoy the advantages of following a renal diet. Instead of a challenging renal regimen, it is a true lifestyle change; the key to starting the diet is to give it adequate attention. Consider living a healthy lifestyle as your goal. Avoid unhealthy snacks, including candies, sugary drinks, frozen foods, and cake-like mixtures.

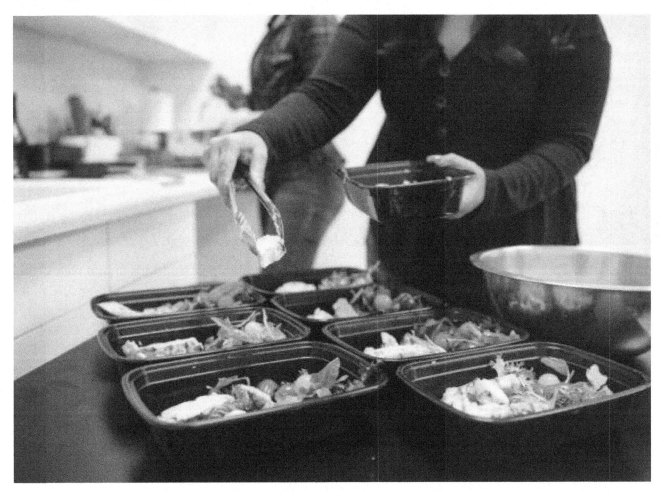

Make sure the pantry doesn't include a lot of fast food. Schedule some time to design a list of food items to buy. A grocery list is a crucial component of shopping that helps to eliminate guessing. Spend some time carefully reading the diet labels and product listings.

## Meal Plan For 28 Days

The purpose of this 28-day meal plan is to reduce some of the uncertainty involved in planning your meals and grocery shopping. For the meal plan balance, you should freeze any chicken broth you make in the first week. If you have leftovers from every meal, substitute them for another dinner or a snack later in the week.

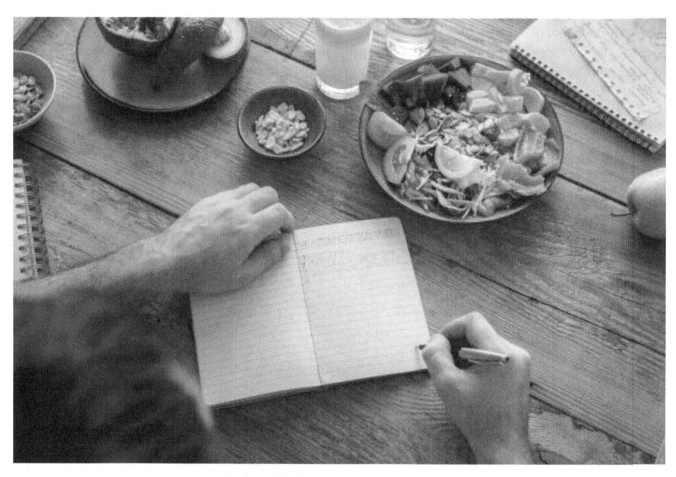

If you need extra protein in your diet, increase the portion sizes of high-protein foods or add high-protein snacks to your diet. The recommended daily protein intake ranges from 35 to 50 grams. To ensure that the specific needs are met, consult a trained dietician.

# Week 1 Meal Plan

**Monday:**

- **Breakfast:** Mixed-Grain Hot Cereal
- **Lunch:** Traditional Chicken-Vegetable Soup
- **Dinner:** Halibut with Lemon Caper Sauce

**Tuesday:**

- **Breakfast:** Corn Pudding
- **Lunch:** Crab Cakes
- **Dinner:** Lamb Chops with Redcurrant and Mint Sauce

**Wednesday:**

- **Breakfast:** Fruit and Cheese Breakfast Wrap
- **Lunch:** Spaghetti with Meat Sauce
- **Dinner:** Baked Tuna

**Thursday:**

- **Breakfast:** Blueberry Muffins
- **Lunch:** Huevos Rancheros
- **Dinner:** Slow-Cooked Lemon Chicken

**Friday:**

- **Breakfast:** Egg-in-the-Hole
- **Lunch:** Vegetarian Reuben Sandwich
- **Dinner:** Simple Salmon Steaks

**Saturday:**

- **Breakfast:** Skillet-Baked Pancake
- **Lunch:** Turkey-Bulgur Soup
- **Dinner:**  Skirt Steak

**Sunday:**

- **Breakfast:** Strawberry–Cream Cheese Stuffed French Toast
- **Lunch:** Moroccan Couscous
- **Dinner:** Chicken Curry

**Suggested Snacks:**

- Veggie Pizza snacks
- Blueberry-Pineapple Smoothie
- Baked eggplant fries.

- Hard-boiled eggs
- Grapes
- Corn Idlis
- 

# Week 2 Meal Plan

**Monday:**

- **Breakfast:** Fruit and Cheese Breakfast Wrap
- **Lunch:** Chicken Curry
- **Dinner:** Classic Pot Roast

**Tuesday:**

- **Breakfast:** Mixed-Grain Hot Cereal
- **Lunch:** Beef Barley Stew
- **Dinner:** Thai Shrimp Kebabs

**Wednesday:**

- **Breakfast**: Blueberry Muffins
- **Lunch:** Fired-Up Zucchini Turkey Burger
- **Dinner:** Persian Chicken

**Thursday:**

- **Breakfast:** Egg-in-the-Hole
- **Lunch:** Taco Stuffing
- **Dinner:** Zesty Orange Tilapia

**Friday:**

- **Breakfast:** Corn Pudding
- **Lunch:** Traditional Chicken-Vegetable Soup
- **Dinner:** Baked Meat Loaf

**Saturday:**

- **Breakfast:** Strawberry–Cream Cheese Stuffed French Toast
- **Lunch:** Pasta Primavera
- **Dinner:** Pesto-Crusted Catfish

**Sunday:**

- **Breakfast:** Skillet-Baked Pancake
- **Lunch:** Broccoli Chicken Casserole
- **Dinner:** Baked Tuna

**Suggested Snacks:**

- Baked Pita chips
- Apple-Chai Smoothie
- Almond Meringue Cookies
- Tuna salad
- Apple
- Unsalted popcorn
- Watermelon

# Week 3 Meal Plan

**Monday:**

- **Breakfast:** Cheesy Scrambled Eggs
- **Lunch:** Eggplant Casserole
- **Dinner:** Chicken Curry

**Tuesday:**

- **Breakfast:** Mixed-Grain Hot Cereal
- **Lunch:** Crab Cakes
- **Dinner:** Baked Meat Loaf

**Wednesday:**

- **Breakfast:** Corn Pudding
- **Lunch:** Veggie Strata
- **Dinner:** Persian Chicken

**Thursday:**

- **Breakfast:** Cinnamon-Nutmeg Blueberry Muffins
- **Lunch:** Hawaiian Chicken Salad
- **Dinner:** Baked Tuna

**Friday:**

- **Breakfast**: Fruit and Cheese Breakfast Wrap
- **Lunch:** Beef Barley Stew
- **Dinner:** Honey Garlic Chicken
- 

**Saturday:**

- **Breakfast:** Beefy Pita Pockets
- **Lunch:** Turkey-Bulgur Soup

- **Dinner:** Chili Rice with Beef

**Sunday:**

- **Breakfast**: Strawberry–Cream Cheese Stuffed French Toast
- **Lunch:** Macaroni and Cheese
- **Dinner:** Halibut with Lemon Caper Sauce

**Suggested Snacks:**

- Grilled Salsa
- Flour Tortilla Chips
- Cornmeal cookies
- Tuna salad
- Jicama and carrots
- Mixed berries
- Buffalo wings

# Week 4 Meal Plan

**Monday:**

- **Breakfast:** Mixed-Grain Hot Cereal
- **Lunch:** Traditional Chicken-Vegetable Soup
- **Dinner:** Halibut with Lemon Caper Sauce

**Tuesday:**

- **Breakfast:** Fruit and Cheese Breakfast Wrap
- **Lunch:** Chicken Curry
- **Dinner:** Classic Pot Roast

**Wednesday:**

- **Breakfast:** Corn Pudding
- **Lunch:** Veggie Strata
- **Dinner:** Persian Chicken

**Thursday:**

- **Breakfast:** Blueberry Muffins
- **Lunch:** Huevos Rancheros
- **Dinner:** Slow-Cooked Lemon Chicken

**Friday:**

- **Breakfast:** Skillet-Baked Pancake

- **Lunch:** Broccoli Chicken Casserole
- **Dinner:** Baked Tuna

## Saturday:

- **Breakfast:** Beefy Pita Pockets
- **Lunch:** Turkey-Bulgur Soup
- **Dinner:** Chili Rice with Beef

## Sunday:

- **Breakfast**: Strawberry–Cream Cheese Stuffed French Toast
- **Lunch:** Macaroni and Cheese
- **Dinner:** Halibut with Lemon Caper Sauce

## Suggested Snacks:

- Baked Pita chips
- Apple-Chai Smoothie
- Almond Meringue Cookies
- Tuna salad
- Apple
- Unsalted popcorn
- Watermelon

## Common Measuring units

There are two widely employed measuring schemes in nutrition: metric and us customary.

| Weight (mass) | |
|---|---|
| **Metric**<br><br>**(grams)** | **US contemporary**<br><br>**(ounces)** |
| 14 grams | 1/2 ounce |
| 28 grams | 1 ounce |
| 85 grams | 3 ounces |
| 100 grams | 3.53 ounces |
| 113 grams | 4 ounces |

| | |
|---|---|
| 227 grams | 8 ounces |
| 340 grams | 12 ounces |
| 454 grams | 16 ounces or 1 pound |

| Volume (liquid) | |
|---|---|
| **Metric** | **US Customary** |
| .6 ml | 1/8 tsp |
| 1.2 ml | 1/4 tsp |
| 2.5 ml | 1/2 tsp |
| 3.7 ml | 3/4 tsp |
| 5 ml | 1 tsp |
| 15 ml | 1 tbsp |
| 30 ml | 2 tbsp |
| 59 ml | 2 fluid ounces or1/4 cup |
| 118 ml | 1/2 cup |
| 177 ml | 3/4 cup |
| 237 ml | 1 cup or 8 fluid ounces |
| 1.9 liters | 8 cups or 1/2 gallon |

| Oven Temperatures | |
|---|---|
| **Metric** | **US contemporary** |
| 121° C | 250° F |
| 149° C | 300° F |
| 177° C | 350° F |
| 204° C | 400° F |
| 232° C | 450° F |

# CHAPTER 4
## Breakfast Recipes

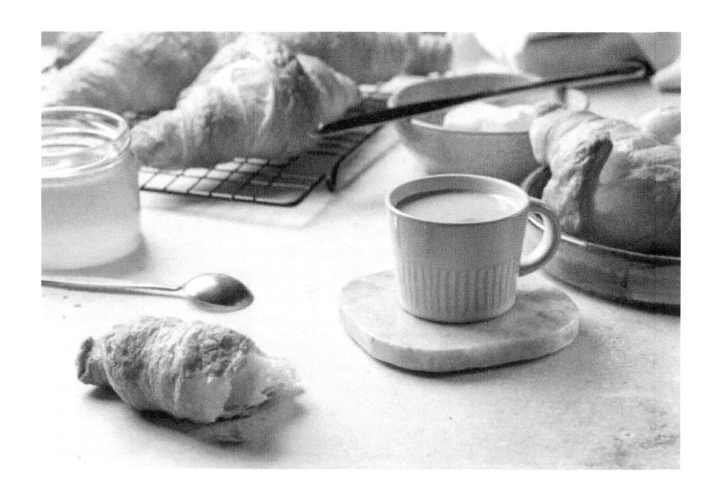

# 1- Strawberry Cream Cheese Stuffed French Toast

Preparation time: 20 minutes

Cooking Time: 65 minutes

Servings: 4

Difficulty Level: Easy

## Nutritional Information:

Calories: 275 kcal, protein: 9 g, carbohydrates: 35 g, Fat: 11 g, Cholesterol: 125 mg, Fiber: 1 g, Sodium: 267 mg, Potassium: 112 mg, Phosphorus: 110 mg, Calcium: 118 mg

## Ingredients:

- ½ cup of plain cream cheese
- Cooking spray for greasing the baking dish
- Eight slices of thick white bread
- 4 tbsp of strawberry jam
- ½ cup of rice milk: unsweetened
- 2 beaten eggs,
- 1 tbsp of sugar: granulated
- ¼ tsp of ground cinnamon
- 1 tsp of vanilla extract

## Instructions:

Preheat the oven to 350°F. Spray an 8-by-8-inch baking dish with cooking spray; set aside. In a small bowl, stir the cream cheese and jam until well blended. Spread 3 tablespoons of the cream cheese mixture onto 4 slices of bread and top with the remaining 4 slices to make sandwiches. Whisk together the eggs, milk, and vanilla in a medium bowl until smooth. Dip the sandwiches into the egg mixture and lay them in the baking dish. Pour any remaining egg mixture over the sandwiches and sprinkle them evenly with sugar and cinnamon. Cover the dish with foil and refrigerate overnight. Bake the French toast, covered, for 1 hour. Remove the foil and bake

for 5 minutes or until the French toast is golden. Serve warm.

# 2- Skillet-Baked Pancake

Preparation time: 15 minutes

Cooking Time: 20 minutes

Servings: 2

Difficulty Level: Easy

## Nutritional Information:

Calories: 201 kcal, protein: 9 g, carbohydrates: 30 g, Fat: 6.5 g, Cholesterol: 186 mg, Fiber: 1 g, Sodium: 83 mg, Potassium: 110 mg, Phosphorus: 167 mg, Calcium: 107 mg

## Ingredients:

- ½ cup of rice milk: unsweetened
- Two eggs
- ¼ tsp of ground cinnamon
- ½ cup of all-purpose flour
- Cooking spray for greasing the skillet
- Pinch of ground nutmeg

## Instructions:

Preheat the oven to 450°F. In a medium bowl, whisk rice milk and eggs. Stir in the cinnamon, nutmeg, and flour until blended but still lumpy (do not overmix). Spray a 9-inch ovenproof pan with cooking spray and put it in the oven for 5 minutes. Take the skillet from the oven carefully and pour batter into the pan. Place the pan in the oven and bake for about 20 minutes until crispy and puffed up on the edges. Split Pancake and serve it.

# 3- Mixed-Grain Hot Cereal

Preparation time: 10 minutes

Cooking Time: 45 minutes

Servings: 2

Difficulty Level: Easy

## Nutritional Information:

Calories: 150 kcal, protein: 5 g, carbohydrates: 30 g, Fat: 1g, Cholesterol: 0 mg, Fiber: 3 g, Sodium: 7 mg, Potassium: 87mg, Phosphorus: 91 mg, Calcium: 15 mg

## Ingredients:

- 1¼ cup of vanilla rice milk
- 2¼ cups of water
- 6 tablespoons of uncooked bulgur
- 1 cup of peeled, sliced apple
- 2 tablespoons of whole buckwheat: uncooked
- ½ teaspoon of ground cinnamon
- 6 tablespoons of plain uncooked couscous

## Instructions:

In a medium saucepan over medium-high heat, heat the water and milk. Boil it, and add the bulgur, buckwheat, and apple. Reduce the heat to low and simmer, occasionally stirring, for 20 to 25 minutes or until the bulgur is tender. Remove the saucepan from the heat and stir in the couscous and cinnamon. Let the saucepan stand for 10 minutes, then fluff the cereal with a fork before serving.

## 4 Fruit and Cheese Breakfast Wrap

Preparation time: 10 minutes

Cooking Time: 0 minutes

Servings: 2

Difficulty Level: Medium

## Nutritional Information:

Calories: 198 kcal, protein: 4 g, carbohydrates: 33g, Fat: 6g, Cholesterol: 16 mg, Fiber: 2 g, Sodium: 200 mg, Potassium: 138 mg, Phosphorus: 79mg, Calcium: 57mg

## Ingredients:

- 2 tablespoons of plain cream cheese
- 2 (6-inch) flour tortillas
- 1 tablespoon of honey
- 1 apple, peeled, cored, and sliced thinly.

## Instructions:

Lay both tortillas on a clean work surface and spread 1 tablespoon of cream cheese onto each tortilla, leaving about ½ inch around the edges. Arrange the apple slices on the cream cheese, just off the center of the tortilla on the side closest to you, leaving about 1½ inches on each side and 2 inches on the bottom. Drizzle the apples lightly with honey. Fold the tortillas' left and right edges into the center, laying the edge over the apples. Fold the tortilla edge closest to you over the fruit and the side pieces. Roll the tortilla away from you, creating a snug wrap. Repeat with the second tortilla.

## 5- Corn Pudding

Preparation time: 10 minutes

Cooking Time: 40 minutes

Servings: 6

Difficulty Level: Medium

## Nutritional Information:

Calories: 180 kcal, protein: 5 g, carbohydrates: 21 g, Fat: 10 g, Cholesterol: 111 mg, Fiber: 6 g, Sodium: 60 mg, Potassium: 198 mg, Phosphorus: 115 mg, Calcium: 59 mg

## Ingredients:

- 1/4 cup sugar
- 1 can of creamed corn
- 1 egg
- 1/4 cup of flour
- 1/4 cup of milk
- 1 dash nutmeg

## Instructions:

Mix sugar, creamed corn, flour, egg, milk, and nutmeg. Spray 9x9''cake Pan. Bake until done, at 350°F. (30 minutes approx.)

## 6- Egg-in-the-Hole

Preparation time: 10 minutes

Cooking Time:  10 minutes

Servings: 2

Difficulty Level: Easy

## Nutritional Information:

Calories: 159 kcal, protein: 9 g, carbohydrates: 15g, Fat: 7g, Cholesterol:213 mg, Fiber: 0.8 g, Sodium: 266mg, Potassium: 122mg, Phosphorus: 137mg, Calcium: 85mg

## Ingredients:

- ¼ cup of unsalted butter
- 2 (½-inch-thick) slices of Italian bread
- Two tablespoons of chopped fresh chives.
- 2 eggs
- Freshly ground black pepper
- Pinch cayenne pepper

## Instructions:

Cut a 2-inch round from the center of each piece of bread using a cookie cutter or a small glass. In a large non-stick skillet over medium-high heat, melt the butter. Place the bread in the skillet, toast it for 1 minute, and then flip it over. Crack the eggs into the holes in the center of the bread and cook for about 2 minutes or until the eggs are set and the bread is golden brown. Top with chopped chives, cayenne pepper, and black pepper. Cook the bread for another 2 minutes. Transfer an egg-in-the-hole to each plate to serve.

## 7- Apple Cinnamon French Toast Strata

Preparation time: 20 minutes

Cooking Time:  50 minutes

Servings: 6-7

Difficulty Level: Medium

## Nutritional Information:

Calories: 324 kcal, protein: 9 g, carbohydrates: 27 g, Fat: 20 g, Cholesterol: 170 mg, Fiber: 1.8 g, Sodium: 280 mg, Potassium: 224 mg, Phosphorus: 150 mg, Calcium: 116 mg

## Ingredients:

- 8 ounces of cream cheese
- 1-pound of cinnamon raisin bread loaf
- 6 tablespoons of unsalted butter
- 1-1/2 medium apples
- 1/4 cup of pancake syrup
- 1 teaspoon of ground cinnamon
- 1-1/4 cup of half & half creamer
- 8 large eggs
- 1-1/4 cup of almond milk, unsweetened

## Instructions:

Dice the cream cheese and bread into cubes. Peel the apples and slice them. Let the butter melt. To coat a 9 x 13 inches baking dish, use the non-stick cooking spray at the bottom of the dish, and place cubed bread. Sprinkle the cubes of cream cheese uniformly over the bread and transfer the apples to the top. Sprinkle the apples with cinnamon and cover the rest of the bread.

Beat the eggs with almond milk, half & half creamer, pancake syrup, and melted butter in a large bowl. Over the bread, pour the mixture. Cover the baking dish with wrap and press down to cover all the pieces. Refrigerate for 2 hours or overnight.

Preheat the oven to 325 ° F. Bake strata for 50 minutes, then let stand for 10 minutes before eating. For 12 servings, split uniformly into squares. Top with pancake, jelly, sugar-free syrup, or applesauce with cinnamon/raspberry if required.

## 8- Bob's Popovers

Preparation time: 10 minutes

Cooking Time: 30 minutes

Servings: 4

Difficulty Level: Easy

### Nutritional Information:

Calories: 82 kcal, protein: 3.4 g, carbohydrates: 11 g, Fat: 2.7 g, Cholesterol: 42 mg, Fiber: 0.3 g, Sodium: 91 mg, Potassium: 66 mg, Phosphorus: 74mg, Calcium: 48mg

### Ingredients:

- 1 cup of 2% milk
- 3 eggs or egg substitute of an equal amount
- 1 cup of white flour
- 1 Tablespoon of sugar
- 1/4 tsp. of salt

### Instructions:

Preheat the oven to 375°F.Put muffin tins in the oven to heat them. Beat the eggs until they are frothy. Be sure to add salt, sugar, oil, and milk. Beat correctly. Add the flour and combine. Remove the muffin tins from the oven and spray them with cooking oil. Fill 3/4 of the cups with batter. Place it in the oven and let it bake for 30 mins. Serve with sugar-free jelly.

## 9- French Toast with Cream Cheese and Applesauce Filling

Preparation time: 10 minutes

Cooking Time: 10 minutes

Servings: 4

Difficulty Level: Medium

### Nutritional Information:

Calories: 276 kcal, protein: 16 g, carbohydrates: 26g, Fat: 12g, Cholesterol:33 mg, Fiber: 5.4 g, Sodium: 466mg, Potassium:314 mg, Phosphorus: 158mg, Calcium: 118mg

### Ingredients:

- 4 tablespoons of egg whites liquid, divided.
- 2 slices of whole-wheat bread
- Two tablespoons of unsweetened applesauce
- cream cheese: 1 ounce
- cinnamon to taste

### Instructions:

On medium heat, preheat a non-stick skillet. Add two tablespoons of egg whites and 1 slice of bread to a bowl. Make sure to get just one side of the bread with the egg. Soak the bread in the egg. In the skillet, put the bread egg side down. Sprinkle with cinnamon and add applesauce and cream cheese to the bread in the pan. For the other slice of bread, repeat step 2 and put it in the pan, egg side up. Brown the other side by turning it as soon as the first bread slice base is browned. Remove and cover with the syrup of your choice.

## 10- Apple Fritter Rings

Preparation time: 10 minutes

Cooking Time: 10 minutes

Servings: 4

Difficulty Level: Easy

### Nutritional Information:

Calories: 145 kcal, protein: 1 g, carbohydrates: 15g, Fat: 9g, Cholesterol: 10 mg, Fiber: 1.3g, Sodium: 33mg, Potassium:67mg, Phosphorus: 26mg, Calcium: 30mg

## Ingredients:

- 1 cup of white flour: all-purpose
- 4 large, tart apples
- 1 teaspoon of baking powder
- 6 tablespoons of sugar (divided use)
- 1/3 cup of 1% low-fat milk
- 1 large egg, beaten.
- 1/3 cup of almond milk
- 1/2 teaspoon of cinnamon
- oil for deep frying, about 3/4 cup
- 1 teaspoon of canola oil

## Instructions:

Peel and cut each apple into 5 rings, each 1/2" thick. Fold the flour, 2 teaspoons of sugar, and baking powder in a mixing bowl. Mix the egg, milk, 1 teaspoon of oil, and almond milk in a separate bowl. To dry ingredients, add egg mixture and stir until just combined. Heat oil to 375º F in a skillet that is 2" deep. In the batter, dip apple slices one at a time. Fried until golden brown in hot oil for around 1-1/2 minutes. Drain on paper towels. Combine the remaining 1/4 cup of cinnamon sugar and scatter on fritters. Serve hot.

## 11- French Toast

Preparation time: 10 minutes

Cooking Time: 35minutes

Servings: 4

Difficulty Level: Easy

## Nutritional Information:

Calories: 218 kcal, protein: 10 g, carbohydrates: 13g, Fat: 14g, Cholesterol:186 mg, Fiber: 2g,

Sodium: 241mg, Potassium:193mg, Phosphorus: 165 mg, Calcium: 167 mg

## Ingredients:

- 1/2 cup of unsalted butter
- 3/4 cup of brown sugar
- 3 tart apples
- 3 teaspoons of cinnamon
- 1/2 cup of dried, sweetened cranberries
- 6 large eggs
- 1 pound loaf of Italian bread
- 1 tablespoon of vanilla
- 1-1/2 cups of rice milk, unenriched

## Instructions:

Scrape, and slice the apples thinly. Combine the melted butter, one teaspoon of cinnamon, and brown sugar in a 13 x 9-inch baking dish. Add cranberries, and Apples are flipped well to cover. Layer the mixture of apples uniformly over the bottom of the baking dish. Cut the bread into 3/4-inch pieces and layer the apples on top. Mix the eggs, vanilla, rice milk, and the remaining 2 teaspoons of cinnamon until well mixed. Pour the paste over the bread and soak the bread entirely. For 4 to 24 hours, cover and refrigerate. Preheat the oven to 375° F. Bake for 30 minutes, wrapped with foil. Uncover the dish and cook for 15 minutes or until the surface turns brown. Remove the dish from the oven and leave it to stay for 5 minutes before cutting it into 9 portions. Serve it warm. Before eating, brush the top with powdered sugar.

## 12- Apple Onion Omelet

Preparation time: 10 minutes

Cooking Time: 25minutes

Servings: 2

Difficulty Level: Easy

## Nutritional Information:

Calories: 284kcal, Protein: 13 g, carbohydrates: 22g, Fat: 16g, Cholesterol:303mg, Fiber: 3.5g, Sodium: 169mg, Potassium:341mg, Phosphorus: 238mg, Calcium: 147mg

## Ingredients:

- 1/4 cup of 1% low-fat milk
- 3 large eggs
- 1/8 teaspoon of black pepper
- 1 tablespoon of water
- 3/4 cup of sweet onion
- 1 tablespoon of butter
- 2 tablespoons of cheddar cheese: shredded
- 1 large apple

## Instructions:

Preheat the oven to 400º F. Peel and thinly cut the apple and onion. Beat the eggs in a small bowl with water, milk, and pepper; set aside. Melt the butter in a small, ovenproof skillet over medium heat. Add the onion and apple to the skillet and fry for around 5 to 6 minutes until the onion becomes translucent.

In the skillet, lay out the onion and apple mixture equally. Pour the egg mixture into the skillet and cook over medium heat until the sides begin to set. Sprinkle with cheddar cheese. Move the skillet to the oven and bake for 10 to 12 minutes until the center is firmly formed. Halve the omelet and slide each half of it onto an individual serving tray.

## 13- Egg Muffins

Preparation time: 10 minutes

Cooking Time: 30 minutes

Servings: 8

Difficulty Level: Easy

## Nutritional Information:

Calories: 154 kcal, protein: 12 g, carbohydrates: 3 g, Fat: 10 g, Cholesterol: 230 mg, Fiber: 0.5g, Sodium: 155mg, Potassium:200 mg, Phosphorus: 154mg, Calcium: 37mg

## Ingredients:

- 1/2 pound of ground beef
- 1 cup of onion
- 1 cup of bell peppers (red, yellow, and orange)
- 1/4 teaspoon of garlic powder
- 1/4 teaspoon of poultry seasoning.
- 1/4 teaspoon of onion powder
- 1/4 teaspoon of salt (optional)
- 1/2 teaspoon of herb seasoning blend
- 8 large eggs
- 1 tablespoon of milk or milk substitute

## Instructions:

Spray with cooking spray on a regular muffin pan, and pre-heat the oven to 350 ° F. Finely slice the onion and bell peppers. Combine the meat, poultry seasoning, onion powder, garlic powder, and herb seasoning to make the sausage in a dish. Cook the sausage crumbles in a non-stick skillet until done, then drain. Mix the milk or milk substitute and salt along with the eggs. Add the sausage crumbles and vegetables and combine. Onto prepared muffin tins, pour the egg mixture, leaving space for muffins to rise. Bake for between 18 to 22 minutes.

## 14 Basic Crepe

Preparation time: 10 minutes

Cooking Time: 30 minutes

Servings: 8

Difficulty Level: Easy

## Nutritional Information:

Calories: 72 kcal, protein: 3 g, carbohydrates: 6 g, Fat: 4 g, Cholesterol: 46 mg, Fiber: 0.1 g,

Sodium: 42 mg, Potassium: 50 mg, Phosphorus: 45 mg, Calcium: 32 mg

## Ingredients:

- 1-1/3 cups of whole milk
- 3 large eggs
- 3 tablespoons of butter, melted.
- 3/4 cup of white flour: all-purpose

## Instructions:

In a processor, blend the eggs and milk to combine. Add the flour slowly and blend for 1 minute. Cover the mixture and let it rest for 1 hour. In a pan, pour crepe batter and whisk in the melted butter. Over a medium-high flame, heat an 8-inch crepe pan or skillet. Cover the pan with butter or spray with non-stick cooking spray. Pour the batter into the pan using a 1/4 cup scale. Make sure that the batter lies equally and, if necessary, move the pan. The crepe is going to bubble mildly. Loose the crepe edges and cut them from the pan until the crepe on the bottom is golden and the edges are finely browned.

## 15- Asparagus and Cheese Crepe Rolls with Parsley

Preparation time: 20 minutes

Cooking Time: 20 minutes

Servings: 4

Difficulty Level: Easy

## Nutritional Information:

Calories: 305kcal, Protein: 10 g, carbohydrates: 16g, Fat: 24 g, Cholesterol:114mg, Fiber: 2.9g, Sodium: 247mg, Potassium: 357mg, Phosphorus: 142mg, Calcium: 96mg

## Ingredients:

- 4 ounces of cream cheese

- 12 asparagus spears
- 1 teaspoon of lemon juice
- 1 bundle of parsley
- 1/2 teaspoon of black pepper
- 1/2 cup of water
- 1/3 cup of all-purpose flour
- 1 egg
- 1/4 cup of cream
- 4 tablespoons of butter
- 2 egg whites

## Instructions:

Steam the asparagus for 10 minutes. Mix cream cheese with lemon juice, spices, and parsley, to make a green cream sauce. Add spices to taste and set aside.

Combine the flour, egg, white water, egg, and 2 tablespoons of melted butter to make crepes; whisk to make a smooth batter. In a skillet (8 to 10-inch crepe or sauté pan), melt 1/2 tablespoon of butter. Add 1/3 cup crepe batter and disperse the batter by rotating the plate. Cook until it is bubbly and the sides start browning. Switch to cook on the other side quickly. On a tray, cool it. To make 4 crepes, repeat with the remaining butter and batter.

Spread the crepes with the stuffing of cream cheese. Distribute the asparagus spears at the end of each crepe equally and fold up tightly into rolls. Roll in foil and allow to cool for one hour in the refrigerator. Before serving, cut the chilled crepes into 3-4 chunks with a sharp knife.

## 16- Asparagus Cauliflower Tortilla

Preparation time: 10 minutes

Cooking Time: 30 minutes

Servings: 4

Difficulty Level: Medium

## Nutritional Information:

Calories: 102 kcal, protein: 9 g, carbohydrates: 9g, Fat: 3g, Cholesterol:0mg, Fiber: 3.88 g, Sodium: 248mg, Potassium:472mg, Phosphorus: 97mg, Calcium: 68mg

## Ingredients:

- 1-1/2 cups of chopped onion,
- 2 cups of chopped cauliflower,
- 1/4 teaspoon of salt
- 2 teaspoons of olive oil
- 1/4 teaspoon of dried thyme leaves: crumbled
- 2 cups of chopped asparagus: bite-size pieces.
- 1 cup of liquid egg substitute: low cholesterol
- 1/4 teaspoon of ground nutmeg
- 1 minced garlic clove.
- 2 tablespoons of finely chopped parsley.
- 1/2 teaspoon of ground pepper

## Instructions:

Place in a microwave-proof, covered dish with asparagus, cauliflower pieces, and one tablespoon of water. Microwave for 3 to 5 minutes, then steam until crisp and tender. Sauté the onion for about 7 minutes until it is golden. Add the garlic and simmer and stir for another 1 minute. Add cauliflower, asparagus, egg substitute, salt, parsley, pepper, nutmeg, and thyme. Decrease heat and cook for 10 to 15 minutes; cover it until set and browned on the bottom. With a knife, remove the sides and invert it onto a heated plate or serve straight from the skillet.

## 17-Raw Apple Cake

Preparation time: 15 minutes

Cooking Time: 1 hour

Servings: 3

Difficulty Level: Easy

## Nutritional Information:

Calories: 340 kcal, protein: 3 g, carbohydrates: 45 g, Fat: 17 g, Cholesterol: 34 mg, Fiber: 1.4 g, Sodium: 164 mg, Potassium: 78 mg, Phosphorus: 53 mg, Calcium: 23 mg

## Ingredients:

- 2 cups of flour
- 1/2 cup of sugar
- 1 cup of cold coffee
- 2 eggs, beaten.
- 1 cup shortening
- 2 tsp. of baking soda
- 1 tsp. of cloves
- 2 tsp. of cinnamon
- 1 cup chopped nuts.
- 2 cups chopped apples.
- 1 cup sour cream
- 3/4 cup raisins

## Instructions:

Grease and flour Baking Sheet of 9 x 13 inches. Preheat the oven to 350 degrees F. Mix in shortening, starch, beaten eggs, baking soda, flour, cinnamon, raisins, cloves, sour cream, sliced apples, cold coffee, and nuts. For 1 hour, bake it. Before serving, cool it.

## 18- Baked Eggs with Basil Pesto

Preparation time: 10 minutes

Cooking Time: 10-15 minutes

Servings: 2

Difficulty Level: Easy

## Nutritional Information:

Calories: 308kcal, Protein: 20.2g, carbohydrates: 7.3g, Fat: 22.1 g, Cholesterol:40mg, Fiber: 1.7g, Sodium: 295mg, Potassium:409mg, Phosphorus: 332mg, Calcium: 33 mg

## Ingredients:

- ½ tsp of Olive Oil
- 2 Eggs, large
- ½ tsp of Lemon juice
- 1-package Basil: 50g, fresh (or use kale)
- ½ tsp of Sunflower seeds, unsalted
- 2 Tbsp of Parmesan cheese, grated.
- ½ tsp of garlic, fresh
- 2 Tbsp of Bell peppers, red, diced.
- ½ Lemon zest
- 2 Tbsp of Zucchini, diced
- ¼ tsp of Cayenne Pepper
- 2 Tbsp of Onions, Spanish, diced

## Instructions:

Use cooking spray to coat the baking dish. Eggs are added to the dish. Cover with vegetables. With cayenne pepper, season it. Bake for 10-15 minutes at 375 degrees F. Meanwhile, make pesto: In the food processor, put olive oil, basil, Parmesan, lemon juice, lemon zest, and sunflower, and combine until the purée forms. Place a spoonful of pesto in the middle when the baked eggs come out of the oven. Serve it.

## 19- Avocado Toast

Preparation time: 5 minutes

Cooking Time: 5 minutes

Servings: 1

Difficulty Level: Easy

## Nutritional Information:

Calories: 174kcal, protein: 3g, carbohydrates: 19 g, Fat: 10g, Cholesterol:6mg, Fiber: 4g, Sodium: 140mg, Potassium:245mg, Phosphorus: 197 mg, Calcium:44mg

## Ingredients:

- 1 pinch of red pepper flakes
- 1/2 avocado mashed or sliced.

- Optional, squeeze fresh lemon or lime.
- 2 slices of gluten-free bread
- 1 pinch of sea salt

## Instructions:

First, toast the bread. Top toasted bread with avocado mashed or sliced. Sprinkle sea salt or red pepper flakes to taste.

## 20- Breakfast Burrito

Preparation time: 10 minutes

Cooking Time: 10 minutes

Servings: 2

Difficulty Level: Easy

## Nutritional Information:

Calories: 366 kcal, protein: 18 g, carbohydrates: 33 g, Fat: 18 g, Cholesterol: 372 mg, Fiber: 2.5 g, Sodium: 594 mg, Potassium: 245 mg, Phosphorus: 300 mg, Calcium: 117 mg

## Ingredients:

- 3 tablespoons of diced Ortega green chiles.
- 4 eggs
- 1/4 teaspoon of ground cumin
- 2 flour tortillas, burrito size
- 1/2 teaspoon of hot pepper sauce
- non-stick cooking spray

## Instructions:

Use non-stick cooking oil to spray a medium-sized skillet and heat it over medium heat. Beat the eggs, hot sauce, cumin, and green chilies in a cup. Pour it into the skillet and cook until the eggs are done; stir for 1 to 2 minutes. Heat the tortillas over medium heat in a microwave or a separate pan for 20 seconds. Put half the egg mixture on each tortilla and roll up burrito style.

## 21- Breakfast Sandwich

Preparation time: 10 minutes

Cooking Time: 10 minutes

Servings: 5-6

Difficulty Level: Easy

### Nutritional Information:

Calories: 253 kcal, protein: 17 g, carbohydrates: 26 g, Fat: 9 g, Cholesterol: 32 mg, Fiber: 2.0 g, Sodium: 591 mg, Potassium: 218 mg, Phosphorus: 158 mg, Calcium: 174 mg

### Ingredients:

- 1 English muffin
- 1/4 cup of liquid egg substitute: low-cholesterol
- 1 tablespoon of shredded cheddar cheese
- 1 turkey sausage patty
- non-stick cooking spray

### Instructions:

Pour the egg substitute into a small skillet sprayed with non-stick cooking spray and cook it on medium-low heat. Turn over with a spatula and cook for 30 seconds until the egg is completely cooked, then toast the English muffin. Put turkey sausage patty on a plate, cover it with a paper towel and cook in the microwave for 1 minute or the period recommended on the box. Place cooked eggs on one toasted piece of English muffin (fold to fit muffin). Cover it with patty sausage, cheddar cheese, and another half of the muffin.

## 22- Breakfast Casserole

Preparation time: 10 minutes

Cooking Time: 55 minutes

Servings: 5-6

Difficulty Level: Medium

### Nutritional Information:

Calories: 224 kcal, protein: 11 g, carbohydrates: 9 g, Fat: 16 g, Cholesterol: 149 mg, Fiber: 0.4 g, Sodium: 356 mg, Potassium: 201 mg, Phosphorus: 159 mg, Calcium: 97 mg

### Ingredients:

- 4 slices of white bread.
- 1 cup of 1% low-fat milk
- 8 ounces pork sausage: reduced-fat.
- 1/2 teaspoon of dry mustard
- 8 ounces of cream cheese
- 1/2 tsp of dried onion flakes
- 5 large eggs

### Instructions:

Preheat the oven to 325° F. Then, cook the sausage in a medium skillet and put it aside. Mix the remaining ingredients in a mixer, except for the bread. Stir in the cooked sausage mixture. Place the pieces of bread in a greased 9" x 9" casserole dish. Pour the mixture of sausages over the bread. Bake until set, or for 55 minutes. Split and serve in 9 pieces.

## 23- Broiled Honey Grapefruit

Preparation time: 5 minutes

Cooking Time: 5 minutes

Servings: 5-6

Difficulty Level: Easy

### Nutritional Information:

Calories: 63 kcal, protein: 1 g, carbohydrates: 17g, Fat: 0g, Cholesterol:0mg, Fiber: 1.2g, Sodium: 1 mg, Potassium:174 mg, Phosphorus: 13mg, Calcium: 20mg

### Ingredients:

- 1 grapefruit
- 1/4 teaspoon of cinnamon
- 2 teaspoons of honey

## Instructions:

Preheat the broiler to 400º F. Slice the grapefruit in half and cut along each section and edge. Sprinkle 1/8 teaspoon of cinnamon and a teaspoon of honey on each half. Broil the grapefruit for six minutes or before the browning begins. Serve it warm.

## 24  Easy Chorizo

Preparation time: 10 minutes

Cooking Time: 10-15 minutes

Servings: 4

Difficulty Level: Easy

## Nutritional Information:

Calories: 155 kcal, protein: 12 g, carbohydrates: 2 g, Fat: 11 g, Cholesterol: 38 mg, Fiber: 1.3 g, Sodium: 97 mg, Potassium: 252 mg, Phosphorus: 114 mg, Calcium: 27 mg

## Ingredients:

- 2 tsp of white vinegar
- 1 tsp of ground oregano
- 2 tbsp of hot chili powder
- 1 pound of 85% lean ground beef
- 3 garlic cloves
- 2 tbsp canola oil
- 2 tsp of cayenne or red pepper
- 1 tsp of black pepper
- 1 tbsp of paprika

## Instructions:

Mince the garlic finely. Mix all ingredients in a large bowl. Place it in an airtight jar and cool it for 12 to 24 hours. Divide the entire recipe into 1/4-cup parts or stock it. Cover them in plastic wrap or butcher paper and freeze them for further use in thick plastic freezer bags. Cook a 1/4-cup portion per person in a non-stick or oiled skillet until ready to eat. With a spatula, chop the beef into fine crumbles.

## 25-  Classic Eggs Benedict

Preparation time: 10 minutes

Cooking Time: 10-15 minutes

Servings: 4

Difficulty Level: Medium

## Nutritional Information:

Calories: 416 kcal, protein: 16 g, carbohydrates: 14 g, Fat: 35 g, Cholesterol: 447 mg, Fiber: 1.05 g, Sodium: 346 mg, Potassium: 174 mg, Phosphorus: 214 mg, Calcium: 105 mg

## Ingredients:

- 2 English muffins
- 3 cups of water (divided use)
- 4 eggs
- 1 tbsp of vinegar
- 1 tbsp of lemon juice
- 1/2 cup of butter: unsalted
- dash of cayenne pepper
- 3 egg yolks
- dash of paprika
- 4 ounces of Canadian bacon, sliced.

## Instructions:

De-mineralize the bacon for 5 minutes by dropping it in 2 cups of boiling water. Remove and put a slotted spoon on top of several paper towels to remove the moisture. Cut the English muffins and toast them. Cut the bacon and put half on each toasted muffin's top.

Combine the vinegar in a large saucepan with about one cup of water. Get it to a boil; lower the flame. Break the eggs one at a time and poach the eggs in the water. Cover and boil for 3-5 minutes or until the eggs are thoroughly cooked. With a slotted spoon, remove the eggs, place them on the top of the bacon and English muffin, wrap it and keep warm. Then melt butter. Beat the yolks of the egg over high heat. Add the cayenne pepper, melted butter, and paprika quickly. Beat until thick with lemon juice. Remove it from the heat and pour it onto the English muffins.

# 26- Egg Tortilla and Chorizo

Preparation time: 5 minutes

Cooking Time: 10-15 minutes

Servings: 2

Difficulty Level: Medium

## Nutritional Information:

Calories: 346kcal, protein: 21g, carbohydrates: 25g, Fat: 18g, Cholesterol:224mg, Fiber: 3.1g, Sodium:316mg, Potassium:397mg, Phosphorus: 278mg, Calcium: 94mg

## Ingredients:

- 2 corn tortillas, 6-inch size
- 1/4 cup of chorizo
- 1 large egg

## Instructions:

Cook a 1/4-cup portion of Quick Chorizo in a pan on top of the stove, and chop the meat with a spatula into fine crumbles. If required, drain the extra fat and water. Add 1 egg until the meat is fully cooked; stir to mix until the egg cooks. With 2 tortillas of corn, serve it.

# 27-Peach Cobbler

Preparation time: 5 minutes

Cooking Time: 3 hours

Servings: 6

Difficulty Level: Medium

## Nutritional Information:

Calories: 150kcal, protein: 1 g, carbohydrates: 23g, Fat: 6g, Cholesterol:15mg, Fiber: 1 g, Sodium:97mg, Potassium:45mg, Phosphorus: 31mg, Calcium: 78mg

## Ingredients:

- ⅔ cup of oats
- 32 ounces peaches: fresh or canned, sliced, and drained.
- ½ cup of butter or margarine: softened.
- ⅔ cup of all-purpose flour
- ½ tsp cinnamon
- ⅔ cup of brown sugar
- ¼ tsp nutmeg

## Instructions:

Put the peaches in a slow cooker. Combine the flour, oats, spices, and sugar in a separate dish. Garnish with butter and mix it until crumbly. Coat peaches with the mixture. Cover and simmer for 3 hours on LOW.

# 28- Cottage Cheese Sour Cream Pancakes

Preparation time: 5 minutes

Cooking Time: 10 minutes

Servings: 4

Difficulty Level: Easy

## Nutritional Information:

Calories: 165kcal, Protein: 8g, carbohydrates: 13g, Fat: 9g, Cholesterol:123mg, Fiber: 0.4g, Sodium:150mg, Potassium:111mg, Phosphorus: 134 mg, Calcium: 64 mg

## Ingredients:

- 1/2 cup of all-purpose flour
- 2 large eggs
- 1/8 teaspoon of salt
- 1/2 cup of sour cream
- 1/2 cup of cottage cheese: small curd

## Instructions:

Slightly beat the eggs. Add whipped cream, cottage cheese, and salt. Mix until combined but not smooth. Fold in the flour gradually. Drop 1/4 cupful onto a hot oiled pan or a non-stick skillet far apart. Cook and brown around the edges until crisp. Turn and brown the other side.

## 29-   Confetti Omelet

Preparation time: 5 minutes

Cooking Time: 10 minutes

Servings: 2

Difficulty Level: Medium

## Nutritional Information:

Calories: 226 kcal, protein: 12g, carbohydrates: 4g, Fat: 1 g, Cholesterol: 203mg, Fiber: 1 g, Sodium:187mg, Potassium:247 mg, Phosphorus: 148 mg, Calcium: 81mg

## Ingredients:

- 2 large eggs
- 1 tbsp canola oil
- 1 tbsp butter
- 2 tbsp orange bell pepper, chopped.
- 4 tbsp 1% low-fat milk
- 2 tbsp fresh mushrooms, sliced.
- 1 tsp garlic, chopped.
- 2 tbsp green onion, chopped.
- 1/8 tsp of ground cumin
- 2 large egg whites
- 1/8 tsps of Pepper
- 2 tbsp of chopped red bell pepper.

## Instructions:

Sauté the vegetables in the butter/oil mixture with garlic until crisp-tender. Eggs, egg whites, and milk are whipped until light and fluffy. Add cumin and pepper to blend. Pour over the sautéed vegetables. Lower the heat and cover for around 1 or 2 minutes. Uncover and raise the sides of the omelet, letting the uncooked egg cook. Fold the omelet in a skillet after the egg is fully cooked. Divide the omelet into 2 pieces and serve instantly. Garnish with a slice of mushroom and green onion.

## 30-   Cran-Apple Oatmeal with Egg

Preparation time: 5 minutes

Cooking Time: 10 minutes

Servings: 2

Difficulty Level: Easy

## Nutritional Information:

Calories: 223kcal, Protein: 10g, carbohydrates: 30g, Fat: 7g, Cholesterol: 212 mg, Fiber: 4g, Sodium:79mg, Potassium:230mg, Phosphorus: 214mg, Calcium: 55mg

## Ingredients:

- 1 small apple, diced.
- 2 tablespoons of dried cranberries
- 2 cups of water
- dash of nutmeg
- 1/4 teaspoon of cinnamon
- 2 large eggs
- 2/3 cup of Oatmeal, quick-cooking

## Instructions:

Mix the water, diced apple or apple sauce, cinnamon, nutmeg, and cranberries in a shallow saucepan. Boil it until the apple is tender, cover, and simmer. Add the Oatmeal, boil, and simmer for 1 minute. Slowly add half of the Oatmeal to the beaten egg, then add that mixture to the Oatmeal and cook it for about 10 seconds. Serve with substituted milk or milk and sweetener, as permitted by the meal schedule.

# 31- Cheesy Scrambled Eggs

Preparation time: 5 minutes

Cooking Time: 5 minutes

Servings: 2

Difficulty Level: Easy

## Nutritional Information:

Calories: 194 kcal, protein: 16 g, carbohydrates: 1 g, Fat: 14 g, Cholesterol: 434 mg, Fiber: 0.2 g, Sodium: 213 mg, Potassium: 192 mg, Phosphorus: 250 mg, Calcium: 214 mg

## Ingredients:

- 1 tablespoon of goat cheese: crumbled
- 2 large eggs
- 1 teaspoon of dried dill weed.
- 1/8 teaspoon of black pepper

## Instructions:

In a cup, beat the eggs; over medium heat, pour them into a non-stick skillet. Eggs are added with black pepper and dill weed. Cook until scrambled. Before serving, top with crumbled goat's cheese.

# 32- Grilled Corn Cakes

Preparation time: 15 minutes

Cooking Time: 10 minutes

Servings: 4

Difficulty Level: Easy

## Nutritional Information:

Calories: 285 kcal, protein: 9 g, carbohydrates: 40 g, Fat: 11 g, Cholesterol: 31 mg, Fiber: 3.7 g, Sodium:409 mg, Potassium:198mg, Phosphorus: 344 mg, Calcium: 234mg

## Ingredients:

- 1/2 teaspoon of anise
- 1 cup of hot water
- 2/3 cup of white corn flour
- Costeño cheese: 4 ounces
- 1 teaspoon of butter

## Instructions:

In a bowl, add the corn flour. Shred the cheese and add it to the flour and add anise. Add hot water; combine with a spatula. Leave for 10 minutes to rest, then knead for 2 to 3 minutes. Form 4 circles of 1/2-inch thick and 4-inches wide to shape the corn cakes. Grease a pan of arepas or skillet. Place each corn cake on the skillet or pan of arepas and cook until lightly browned.

# 33- Denver Omelet

Preparation time: 10 minutes

Cooking Time: 5 minutes

Servings: 2

Difficulty Level: Easy

## Nutritional Information:

Calories: 228 kcal, protein: 17 g, carbohydrates: 7 g, Fat: 15 g, Cholesterol: 233 mg, Fiber: 0.9 g, Sodium: 360 mg, Potassium: 275 mg, Phosphorus: 226 mg, Calcium: 142 mg

## Ingredients:

- 1 large egg
- 1/2-ounce of ham
- 1/4 cup of onion
- 1 teaspoon of canola oil

- 1/4 cup of bell pepper
- 1/2-ounce of cheddar cheese, shredded.
- 1 egg white

## Instructions:

Dice the onion, ham, and bell pepper. Heat oil on medium heat. Add the onion, ham, and pepper to a pan. For 2 minutes, sauté. Beat the egg and the egg white. Pour the mixture into the skillet. Cook and then use a spatula to remove the omelet. On a serving tray, fold it over and scatter cheese on it.

## 34  Vegetables Omelet

Preparation time: 10 minutes

Cooking Time: 10-15 minutes

Servings: 2

Difficulty Level: Easy

## Nutritional Information:

Calories: 187kcal, protein: 22g, carbohydrates: 12g, Fat: 6g, Cholesterol: 215mg, Fiber: 2.2g, Sodium:270mg, Potassium:352mg, Phosphorus: 218mg, Calcium: 165 mg

## Ingredients:

- 1 large egg
- 1/4 cup of whole kernel corn, thawed.
- non-stick cooking spray
- 1/3 cup of zucchini, chopped.
- 2 tbsp water
- 1-ounce cheddar cheese, low-fat shredded
- 3 tbsp of green onion, chopped.
- 1/4 tsp of Extra Spicy herb seasoning blend
- 2 large egg whites

## Instructions :

Over a medium-high flame, warm a small saucepan and spray cooking oil. Add the zucchini, onions, and corn to the pan; simmer for 4 minutes or until the vegetables are tender and crisp. Carefully remove from the heat. Over medium-high heat, warms a 10" non-stick skillet. Mix egg, whites, pepper, and water in a cup, stirring well. Coat pan with cooking spray. Pour the mixture of eggs into the pan; cook until the edges appear to set (about 2 minutes). Use the spatula to softly raise the omelet's sides and tilt the pan to cook the uncooked egg mixture.

Spoon the vegetable mixture over half of the omelet and scatter the cheese over the vegetable mixture. Then fold the omelet in half with a spatula. Cook for an additional 2 minutes or before the cheese melts. Slide the omelet cautiously onto a pan.

## 35- Raised Waffles.

Preparation time: 10 minutes

Cooking Time: 20 minutes

Servings: 6

Difficulty Level: Medium

## Nutritional Information:

Calories: 222kcal, protein:5g, carbohydrates: 30g, Fat: 9g, Cholesterol:53mg, Fiber: 1.5 g, Sodium:78mg, Potassium: 109mg, Phosphorus: 96 mg, Calcium: 13mg

## Ingredients:

- 2 cups of rice drink: non-dairy unenriched
- 1/2 cup of warm water
- 1/4 cup of canola oil
- dry active yeast: 2 envelopes
- 1/8 tsp salt
- 2 eggs, beaten lightly.
- 1 tsp sugar
- 1-1/2 cup of white flour

## Instructions:

Add yeast and water to a wide mixing bowl, stir it to dissolve, and set it for 5 mins. Add rice drink, salt, sugar, and oil. Beat cornmeal, flour, and eggs; do not beat too much. Let the mixture set in a warm place for about 15 mins until it rises. Use a preheated waffle iron for cooking. Split the cooked waffle into 2-square pieces and top it with fresh fruit or syrup.

## 36-  Blueberry Muffins

Preparation time: 10 minutes

Cooking Time: 30 minutes

Servings: 6

Difficulty Level: Easy

### Nutritional Information:

Calories: 250 kcal, protein: 10 g, carbohydrates: 30 g, Fat: 10 g, Cholesterol:31mg, Fiber: 1.3g, Sodium:178mg, Potassium:136 mg, Phosphorus: 85mg, Calcium: 55 mg

### Ingredients:

- 3/4 cup of brown sugar
- 1 cup of fresh blueberries
- 1 cup of rolled oats.
- 1/2 cup of olive oil
- 1 cup of plain Greek yogurt: nonfat
- 1/2 tsp of cream of tartar
- 1/4 cup of water
- 1 large egg
- 1 cup of all-purpose flour
- 1/2 tsp salt
- 1-1/3 cups of whey protein powder
- 1/2 tsp of baking soda

### Instructions:

Preheat the oven to 350° F. Mix the oats with yogurt in a large bowl, add egg, water, oil, and sugar, and blend well. In a separate bowl,

combine protein powder, flour, salt, tartar cream, and baking soda. Mix all dried ingredients with wet ingredients and add blueberries. Grease 12 muffin cups or muffin pans and add the batter to them. Bake for 20 to 25 minutes.

## 37-Maple Pancakes

Preparation time: 10 minutes

Cooking Time: 10 minutes

Servings: 5

Difficulty Level: Easy

### Nutritional Information:

Calories: 178 kcal, protein: 6 g, carbohydrates: 25 g, Fat: 6 g, Cholesterol: 2 mg, Fiber: 0.7 g, Sodium: 297 mg, Potassium: 126 mg, Phosphorus: 116 mg, Calcium: 174 mg

### Ingredients:

- 2 large egg whites
- 1 tbsp maple extract
- 1 cup of all-purpose flour
- 2 tsp baking powder
- 1 tbsp granulated sugar
- 1/8 tsp salt
- 2 tbsp canola oil
- 1 cup of 1% low-fat milk

### Instructions :

Combine the sugar, flour, salt, and baking powder in a medium mixing dish, and center of the dry mixture, create a well. Now combine milk, maple extract, egg whites, and oil in a separate large mixing bowl. Add egg mixture into the dry mixture all at once. Stir until fully moistened (batter should be lumpy). Pour around 1/4 cup batter onto a hot, finely greased griddle to create 4" pancakes. Cook each side for around 2 minutes over medium heat. When the top is bubbly and the sides are partially crisp, turn the Pancake. Avoid pressing with the spatula to keep the pancakes light and fluffy.

# 38- Hazelnut Cinnamon Coffee

Preparation time: 10 minutes

Cooking Time: 0 minutes

Servings: 4

Difficulty Level: Easy

## Nutritional Information:

Calories: 13kcal, protein:1 g, carbohydrates: 1g, Fat: 0 g, Cholesterol:1mg, Fiber: 0 g, Sodium:13mg, Potassium: 139mg, Phosphorus: 22mg, Calcium: 24 mg

## Ingredients:

- 8 tsp Classic Hazelnut Syrup: Sugar-Free
- 4 cups of brewed coffee.
- 4 cinnamon sticks
- 4 tbsp1% low-fat milk

## Instructions:

Use the coffee maker to brew coffee. Pour it into small cups. Add in each mug 1 tablespoon milk and 2 teaspoons Sugar-Free Classic Hazelnut Syrup, and garnish each with a stick of cinnamon.

# 39- Almond Milk

Preparation time: 10 minutes ( 6 hours refrigeration time)

Cooking Time: 0 minutes

Servings: 2

Difficulty Level: Easy

## Nutritional Information:

Calories: 40kcal, protein: 1 g, carbohydrates: 2g, Fat: 3g, Cholesterol 0mg, Fiber: 0.6g, Sodium:9.6mg, Potassium:37mg, Phosphorus: 30mg, Calcium: 120mg

## Ingredients:

- 3 cups of filtered water and water for soaking.
- 1 tsp of vanilla extract
- 1 cup of raw almonds

## Instructions:

Add the raw almonds and filtered water to the container and cover it. Soak in the refrigerator for 6 hours at room temperature or overnight. Drain the almonds, then add them to a mixer with three cups of filtered water.

Blend on a low level and then on a high setting. Blend until the almonds are finely sliced, and the mixture turns white. Pour the liquid into a bowl using a cheesecloth to strain the liquid from the batches' almond meal. Discard the almond meal. Use flavorings of choice or vanilla extract, and serve it cool.

# 40- Ginger-Apple Sparkler

Preparation time: 10 minutes

Cooking Time: 1 hour

Servings: 6

Difficulty Level: Medium

## Nutritional Information:

Calories: 185 kcal, protein: 0 g, carbohydrates: 47 g, Fat: 0 g, Cholesterol: 0 mg, Fiber: 0.3 g, Sodium: 25 mg, Potassium: 110 mg, Phosphorus: 7 mg, Calcium: 7 mg

## Ingredients:

- 12 pieces of crystallized ginger.
- 2 cups of sugar
- 2 cups of water

- 1 six-inch piece of finely diced fresh ginger.
- 4 cups of sparkling apple cider.
- ice cubes
- 6 cinnamon sticks: cut half.

## Instructions:

Add water, sugar, and grated ginger to a saucepan to make ginger syrup and boil it. Lower the heat and simmer for 1 hour until the ginger taste is strong. Strain the mixture and cool it. Then add one tablespoon of ginger syrup to each bottle to prepare the Ginger-Apple Sparkler.Add1/2 cup of cider and ice cubes; mix it. Use crystallized ginger or cinnamon stick for garnishing.

## 41- Green Beans with Turnips

Preparation time: 5 minutes

Cooking Time: 15 minutes

Servings: 4

Difficulty Level: Medium

## Nutritional Information:

Calories: 58 kcal, protein: 1 g, carbohydrates: 7 g, Fat: 3 g, Cholesterol: 8 mg, Fiber: 3.0 g, Sodium: 104 mg, Potassium: 199 mg, Phosphorus: 33 mg, Calcium: 36 mg

## Ingredients:

- 2 turnips: medium
- fresh green beans: 1-pound
- 1 tbsp butter: unsalted
- 2 garlic cloves
- 1/4 tsp paprika
- 1/4 tsp salt
- 1/2 tsp black pepper

## Instructions:

Strip the green beans from the ends and break into 1-1/2" pieces. Peel turnips and cut 8 pieces of each. Mince the garlic. Put a medium-size pot with vegetables and garlic. Cover and bring to a boil with 3 cups of water. Reduce heat to medium and cook for 15 minutes uncovered. Remove the pot from the heat and drain the water. Add salt, pepper, and butter. To combine seasonings with vegetables, toss gently and sprinkle paprika. Serve warm.

## 42- Fresh Fruit Compote

Preparation time: 5 minutes(Refrigeration time: 4 hours)

Cooking Time: 0 minutes

Servings: 4

Difficulty Level: Medium

## Nutritional Information:

Calories: 44 kcal, protein:0.5g, carbohydrates: 11g, Fat: 0.2 g, Cholesterol: 0mg, Fiber: 1.6g, Sodium:1mg, Potassium:140mg, Phosphorus: 13mg, Calcium: 32mg

## Ingredients:

- 1 Banana: bite-size pieces.
- 1/4 cup of red raspberries, sweetened.
- 1/2 cup of Peaches, cut.
- 1/2 cup of Strawberries,
- 1/2 cup of Orange juice, unsweetened
- 1 Apple: bite-size pieces.
- 1/2 cup of Blackberries,
- 1/2 cup of Blueberries,

## Instructions:

Add low-fat orange juice and all the mentioned ingredients to a huge bottle. Gently shake it. Give four hours at room temp to thaw by using frozen berries.

## 43- Shrimp Tacos

Preparation time: 30 minutes

Cooking Time: 10 minutes

Servings: 4

Difficulty Level: Medium

### Nutritional Information:

Calories: 394kcal, protein: 19g, carbohydrates: 30g, Fat: 22g, Cholesterol: 134 mg, Fiber: 4.2g, Sodium:235mg, Potassium:392mg, Phosphorus: 335mg, Calcium: 177mg

### Ingredients:

- 2 limes
- 1/2 tsp of ground cumin
- 12 corn tortillas: 6-inch size
- 1/2 tsp chili powder
- 1-1/2 cups of shredded cabbage.
- 1/2 cup of mayonnaise
- 1/2 bunch cilantro
- 2 tbsp milk
- 1 garlic clove
- 2 tbsp olive oil
- 1/4 cup of sour cream
- 1/2 cup of red onion
- 1-pound raw shrimp, fresh, medium-size

### Instructions:

Shred cabbage, cut cilantro and onion, and mince the garlic. Devein and shell shrimp, put it in a dish, and squeeze lime juice over the shrimp. Sprinkle curry powder, cumin, 1 tablespoon of olive oil, and chopped garlic over it. Marinate and cool for 15 to 30 minutes.

Add half the lime juice to mayonnaise, milk, and sour cream to make Salsa Blanca. Stir to mix and cool it in the refrigerator. Heat the remaining 1 tablespoon of olive oil in a wide skillet over medium to high heat and add shrimp; Cook for 2 to 4 minutes until shrimp is done.

Take out shrimp from the saucepan when it turns pink. Do not overcook. Cook the corn tortillas in a pan, one by one, until they are soft. To keep them warm, cover them in a clean dishtowel. Place 4 shrimp on each tortilla to assemble the tacos and top with cilantro, salsa Blanca, lime wedges, cabbage, and red onion. If needed, add hot sauce.

## 44  Mexican Egg & Tortilla Skillet Breakfast

Preparation time: 10 minutes

Cooking Time: 10 minutes

Servings: 6

Difficulty Level: Medium

### Nutritional Information:

Calories: 297kcal, protein:11g, carbohydrates: 20g, Fat: 20g, Cholesterol: 199mg, Fiber: 2g, Sodium:267mg, Potassium: 152mg, Phosphorus: 179mg, Calcium: 148mg

### Ingredients:

- 2 green onions thinly sliced.
- 1/4 cup ketchup: low salt
- 1 bag (6oz) tortilla chips: unsalted, broken up.
- 1 tsp chili powder
- 2 Tbsp Butter
- 8 eggs

### Instructions:

Whisk the eggs until they are thoroughly combined. Add onion, ketchup, and chili powder. Beat it until well blended. In a pan, melt the butter, add tortilla chips and fry until warmed through, on moderate heat. Pour the mixture of eggs and cook until the perfect consistency is reached. Serve hot. (You can use flour tortillas and split them into fourths if you cannot find unsalted tortilla chips. Bake until crisp at 350°F)

## 45- Apple Peanut Butter Cookies

Preparation time: 10 minutes

Cooking Time: 10-15 minutes

Servings: 2 ½ dozen

Difficulty Level: Medium

### Nutritional Information:

Calories: 108kcal, protein:2g, carbohydrates: 13g, Fat: 6g, Cholesterol: 6mg, Fiber: 1g, Sodium:85mg, Potassium:68mg, Phosphorus: 56mg, Calcium: 40 mg

### Ingredients:

- 1/2 cup of Peanut Butter
- 1/2 cup of Shortening.
- 1/2 cup of Sugar
- 1 egg
- 1/2 cup of Packed Brown Sugar
- 1 1/2 cup of All-Purpose Flour
- 1/2 tsp. of Vanilla Extract
- 1/2 tsp. of Salt
- 1/2 tsp. of Baking Soda
- 1 cup of an apple peeled and grated.
- 1/2 tsp. of Ground Cinnamon

### Instructions:

Cream the sugar, shortening, and peanut butter in a wide bowl until light and fluffy. Whisk in the vanilla and egg. Mix the dry ingredients; slowly add to the creamed mixture and mix properly. Add apple. Place 2 inches apart on greased baking sheets with rounded tablespoonfuls. Bake for 10-12 minutes at 375°F or until golden brown. Before removing from wire racks, cool for 5 minutes.

## 46- Low Sodium Pound Cake

Preparation time: 10 minutes

Cooking Time: 30 minutes

Servings: 5-6

Difficulty Level: Easy

### Nutritional Information:

Calories:243 kcal, protein: 3.7 g, carbohydrates: 31 g, Fat: 12 g, Cholesterol: 75 mg, Fiber: 0.6 g, Sodium: 18 mg, Potassium: 47 mg, Phosphorus: 45 mg, Calcium: 30 mg

### Ingredients:

- 3/4 cup of Sugar
- 2 large eggs, beaten slightly.
- 1 1/4 cup of bread flour
- 3 oz. of Milk
- 1/4 lb. of butter, unsalted

### Instructions:

Beat butter and sugar until creamy and fluffy. Add milk, eggs, and flour and mix thoroughly. Use pan paper to line the 18×13-inch pan. Bake for 30 minutes at 375-degree F.

## 47-Tuna Sandwich

Preparation time: 10 minutes

Cooking Time: 10-15 minutes

Servings: 2

Difficulty Level: Easy

### Nutritional Information:

Calories:29 kcal, protein: 24g, carbohydrates:30g, Fat: 10g, Cholesterol: 30mg, Fiber: 2g, Sodium:520mg, Potassium:160mg, Phosphorus: 120mg, Calcium: 20 mg

### Ingredients:

- 7 ounces of low-sodium: canned, water-packed tuna.
- 1 tsp of herb seasoning blend
- 5 large eggs

- 1/4 cup of onion
- 4 lemon slices
- 1 tsp of turmeric
- 1/2 cup of fresh cilantro
- 1 garlic clove
- 4 pita bread, 6-inch size
- 1/2 tsp of lemon pepper seasoning salt-free
- 1/4 cup of canola oil

## Instructions:

Cut the onion, garlic, and cilantro. In a bowl, put all the ingredients, except the oil. Mix until it is combined properly. Heat oil over a moderate flame in a pan. To form one wide patty, spoon the tuna paste into the pan. Fry until brown and crispy golden, turning once. Cut the tuna patty into four equal sections. Serve with a lemon wedge and pita bread.

## 48- Cereal with Cranberry-Orange Twist

Preparation time: 5 minutes

Cooking Time: 5 minutes

Servings: 2

Difficulty Level: Easy

## Nutritional Information:

Calories:120kcal, protein:4g, carbohydrates:19g, Fat: 4 g, Cholesterol: 190mg, Fiber: 2 g, Sodium:70 mg, Potassium:85.9mg, Phosphorus: 76mg, Calcium: 90 mg

## Ingredients:

- ½ cup of water
- 1/4 cup of dried cranberries
- ½ cup of orange juice
- 1/3 cup of oat bran

## Instructions:

Combine all ingredients in a bowl. Microwave the bowl for about 2 minutes and serve with milk and sugar. Also, you can add honey. Enjoy!

## 49- Banana Oat Shake

Preparation time: 10 minutes

Cooking Time: 0 minutes

Servings: 1-2

Difficulty Level: Easy

## Nutritional Information:

Calories:203kcal, protein:6 g, carbohydrates: 33g, Fat: 2.4g, Cholesterol: 3.7 mg, Fiber: 3 g, Sodium:195mg, Potassium:52mg, Phosphorus: 1 mg, Calcium: 128.2mg

## Ingredients:

- 2/3 cup of skim milk
- 1/2 cup of cooked Oatmeal, chilled
- 1/2 of frozen banana: chunks.
- 2 tbsp brown sugar
- 1 1/2 tbsp vanilla extract
- 1 tbsp wheat germ

## Instructions:

In a blender, put the Oatmeal and process for a few mins. Add brown sugar, milk, vanilla, wheat germ, and 1/2 banana mixture. Blend until smooth and dense. If needed, serve with ice.

## 50- Beefy Pita Pockets

Preparation time: 10 minutes

Cooking Time: 15-20 minutes

Servings: 3-4

Difficulty Level: Easy

## Nutritional Information:

Calories:421kcal, protein:21g, carbohydrates:37g, Fat: 21g, Cholesterol: 57mg, Fiber: 3g, Sodium:393mg, Potassium:443mg, Phosphorus: 193mg, Calcium: 102mg

## Ingredients:

- 1 onion: medium
- 2 tbsp olive oil
- 1 red bell pepper: medium
- 2 cups of mushrooms
- 1 tbsp Worcestershire sauce
- 1/2 cup of parsley
- 1-pound lean ground beef
- 1 tbsp of browning and seasoning sauce
- 6 pieces of pita bread
- 1/2 tsp black pepper

## Instructions:

Cut the onion and mushrooms into small strips; slice the bell pepper. Parsley chop. Heat the olive oil over medium-high heat in a large skillet. Add bell pepper, onion, and mushroom. Sauté for around 6 minutes, until the vegetables are soft. Place the vegetables on a tray. Then add beef to the skillet; cook for 5 to 6 minutes until no sign of pink remains. Spoon off the fat and dispose of it. Add the Worcestershire sauce, black pepper, and Kitchen Bouquet sauce; mix and simmer for 1 to 2 minutes. Add vegetables and stir to mix. Stir in the parsley and simmer until the mixture is hot. Switch from heat. Then warm Pitas. Cut off each pita's side with a 2" strip, pull it open, and fill each pita's beef and vegetable mixture.

## 51- High Protein Bread

Preparation time: 40 minutes

Cooking Time: 60 minutes

Servings: 6

Difficulty Level: Medium

## Nutritional Information:

Calories:47kcal, protein:2.3g, carbohydrates:8.32g, Fat: 0.42g, Cholesterol: 1mg, Fiber: 0.6g, Sodium:77mg, Potassium:61mg, Phosphorus: 35mg, Calcium: 24mg

## Ingredients:

- 1 cup of all-purpose flour
- 3 cups of whole wheat flour
- 1/2 cup of wheat gluten
- 1/2 tsp salt
- 2 tbsp sugar
- 1/3 cup of honey
- 2 tbsp yeast
- 2 cups of warm water, 95-105 degrees
- 1 1/2 tsp of canola oil

## Instructions:

In a mixing bowl, combine the sugar, flour, and gluten. Mix the oil, yeast, and honey into the water in a separate bowl. Let stand and swirl for around 5 minutes until the yeast is dissolved. To make the dough, add the yeast mixture to the flour mix. Knead the dough until the texture is elastic, adding more flour if required to the board. This usually requires about 5 minutes. Cover the dough with a towel in a clean, lightly oiled container. Let it rest until its size doubles. Depending on the heat and humidity, this could take 45 minutes to an hour.

Preheat the oven to 350 degrees F and spray the oil on your 5×9-inch pan. Punch the dough down and arrange it in a pan. Let it rise to the top of the pan again. This could take from 30 minutes to an hour,

The bread should be dark brown and in the oven for 50-55 minutes. It should have an internal temperature of about 200 degrees F and sound hollow on tapping. After it has cooled, extract the loaf from the pan. Until slicing, let the loaf cool on a rack.

## 52- Overnight Oatmeal

Preparation time: 10 minutes

Cooking Time: 7-8 hours

Servings: 6-8

Difficulty Level: Medium

### Nutritional Information:

Calories: 209kcal, protein:7g, carbohydrates: 29 g, Fat: 7g, Cholesterol: 8mg, Fiber: 3g, Sodium:64 mg, Potassium:214mg, Phosphorus: 176mg, Calcium: 205mg

### Ingredients:

- 1 tsp of cinnamon
- 8 cups of water
- ⅓ cup of dried cranberries
- 2 cups of steel-cut oats

### Instructions:

Spray cooking oil inside a slow cooker. Combine a 5-quart slow cooker with water, dried cranberries, and oats. Cover and simmer until the oats are soft and the porridge is fluffy, on LOW for 7-8 hours.

## 53- Strawberry Bread

Preparation time: 10 minutes

Cooking Time: 60 minutes

Servings: 8

Difficulty Level: Easy

### Nutritional Information:

Calories: 254 kcal, protein: 3 g, carbohydrates: 33 g, Fat: 12 g, Cholesterol: 42 mg, Fiber: 0.8 g, Sodium: 157 mg, Potassium: 64 mg, Phosphorus: 39 mg, Calcium: 10 mg

### Ingredients:

- 2 cups of sugar
- 3 cups of flour
- 1 tsp. of baking soda
- 1/2 cup of oil
- 1 tsp. of salt (or 1/2tsp)
- 4 eggs (beaten)
- 1/2 cup of apple sauce
- 1 tsp. of vanilla
- 20 oz. strawberries (sweetened)

### Instructions:

Mix dry ingredients (sugar, flour, salt, soda).In the middle, create a well. Mix the liquids (applesauce, oil, eggs, vanilla, strawberries) in a separate bowl and pour it into a well. Mix all by hand, keeping the strawberries partly intact. No need for over-mixing. Put in 2 pans that are greased or in a Bundt pan. Bake for one hour at 350°F.

## 54  Coconut Bread

Preparation time: 20 minutes

Cooking Time: 60 minutes

Servings: 6-8

Difficulty Level: Medium

### Nutritional Information:

Calories:258kcal, protein:4g, carbohydrates:29g, Fat: 14g, Cholesterol: 54mg, Fiber: 0.9g, Sodium:204mg, Potassium:82 mg, Phosphorus: 73mg, Calcium: 61mg

### Ingredients:

- 1/3 cup of unsalted butter
- 2 tbsp of coconut oil
- 1/2 cup of sugar
- 1 cup of dried, shredded coconut: sweetened.
- 2 large eggs
- 1 cup of sour cream
- 1 tsp baking soda

- 2 cups of all-purpose flour
- 1-1/2 tsp baking powder.

## Instructions:

Preheat the oven to 350° F. Grease a pan of 9 x 5-inch. Set out the butter to soften it. In the oven, heat the coconut oil until it melts. Left to cool aside. Cream together the butter and sugar. Add coconut oil and eggs; whisk together, then add sour cream. To blend, add the shredded coconut and swirl.

Mix the rice, baking powder, and baking soda in a separate dish. Then combine dry ingredients with egg mixture, pour it into greased loaf pan and bake until the knife inserted inside comes clean. Cool it to serve in breakfast.

## 55- Dilly Scrambled Eggs

Preparation time: 5 minutes

Cooking Time: 10 minutes

Servings: 2

Difficulty Level: Easy

## Nutritional Information:

Calories:194 kcal, protein:16g, carbohydrates:1g, Fat: 14 g, Cholesterol: 434mg, Fiber: 0.2 g, Sodium:213mg, Potassium:192mg, Phosphorus: 250mg, Calcium: 214mg

## Ingredients:

- 1/8 teaspoon of black pepper
- 2 large eggs
- 1 tablespoon of crumbled goat cheese
- 1 teaspoon of dried dill weed

## Instructions:

The eggs are beaten in a bowl before being added to a nonstick pan over medium heat. To eggs, add dill weed & black pepper. Scramble the

eggs after cooking them. Before serving, sprinkle goat cheese crumbles over the top.

## 56- Apple Oatmeal Custard

Preparation time: 5 minutes

Cooking Time: 5-10 minutes

Servings: 1

Difficulty Level: Easy

## Nutritional Information:

Calories:248kcal, protein:11g, carbohydrates:33g, Fat: 8g, Cholesterol: 186 mg, Fiber: 5.8g, Sodium:164mg, Potassium:362 mg, Phosphorus: 240 mg, Calcium: 154 mg

## Ingredients:

- 1/3 cup of quick-cooking oatmeal
- 1/2 medium apple
- 1 large egg
- 1/4 teaspoon of cinnamon
- 1/2 cup of almond milk

## Instructions:

Apples are halved, cored, and finely chopped. In a big mug, mix oats, egg, & almond milk. With a fork, stir well. Add apple with cinnamon. Stir till combined. For 2 minutes on high in a microwave, cook it. With a fork, fluff it. If necessary, cook for an additional 30 to 60 seconds. If you want your cereal to be thinner, stir in a little more milk or water.

## 57- Breakfast Bagel

Preparation time: 5 minutes

Cooking Time: 5 minutes

Servings: 1

Difficulty Level: Easy

## Nutritional Information:

Calories: 134 kcal, protein: 5 g, carbohydrates: 19 g, Fat: 6 g, Cholesterol: 15 mg, Fiber: 1.6 g, Sodium: 219 mg, Potassium: 162 mg, Phosphorus: 50 mg, Calcium: 9mg

## Ingredients:

- 2 tablespoons of cream cheese
- 1 bagel; 2-ounce size
- 2 tomato slices; 1/4-inch thick
- 1 teaspoon of lemon pepper seasoning; low-sodium
- 2 red onions; sliced

## Instructions:

Bagel is sliced and toasted till golden. Each bagel half is covered with cream cheese. Slices of tomato & onion are placed on top; then lemon pepper is sprinkled.

## 58- Asian Pear Crisp

Preparation time: 20 minutes

Cooking Time: 50 minutes

Servings: 6-8

Difficulty Level: Medium

## Nutritional Information:

Calories:401kcal, protein:6g, carbohydrates:56 g, Fat: 10g, Cholesterol: 23mg, Fiber: 5 g, Sodium:53mg, Potassium:127mg, Phosphorus: 86mg, Calcium: 45mg

## Ingredients:

- 1/2 cup of unbleached all-purpose flour
- 3/4 cup of nuts, chopped
- 4 tablespoons of granulated sugar; divided
- 1/4 cup of light brown sugar
- 1/4 teaspoon of ground cinnamon

- 5 tablespoons of unsalted butter
- 1/8 teaspoon of ground nutmeg
- 1 tablespoon of cornstarch
- 3 pounds of Asian pears; peeled & core
- juice of one lemon

## Instructions:

Set oven to 375 degrees Fahrenheit. In a food processor, combine the nuts, flour, brown sugar, two tbsp of granulated sugar, cinnamon, & nutmeg. Blend the ingredients with melted butter until it resembles wet sand. In a large bowl, combine the remaining two tbsp of granulated sugar, cornstarch, & lemon juice. Pears are peeled before being cut in half and cored. Slice first into wedges, then in half. Pears are tossed with the sugar mixture and placed in an 8-inch baking dish. Add topping to the pears. Bake for approximately 45 minutes until the topping is deeply golden brown and fruit is bubbling around the edges. Cool for approximately 15 minutes on a wire rack, Serve.

## 59- Chicken N' Orange Salad Sandwich

Preparation time: 10 minutes

Cooking Time: 0 minutes

Servings: 6

Difficulty Level: Medium

## Nutritional Information:

Calories: 162 kcal, protein: 12 g, carbohydrates:6g, Fat: 10 g, Cholesterol: 52mg, Fiber: 10 g, Sodium:93mg, Potassium:241mg, Phosphorus: 106mg, Calcium: 13 mg

## Ingredients:

- 1/2 cup of green pepper; chopped
- 1 cup of chopped cooked chicken
- 1/4 cup of onion; finely sliced
- 1/2 cup of celery, diced
- 1/3 cup of mayonnaise

- 1 cup of Mandarin oranges

Mix chicken, green pepper, celery, and onion. Mayonnaise and mandarin oranges are added. Mix thoroughly. On bread, spread it and serve it.

## 60- Black Bean Burger

Preparation time: 10 minutes

Cooking Time: 20 minutes

Servings: 4

Difficulty Level: Medium

### Nutritional Information:

Calories: 398kcal, protein:16 g, carbohydrates:40g, Fat: 20 g, Cholesterol: 20mg, Fiber: 10g, Sodium:371mg, Potassium:444mg, Phosphorus: 160mg, Calcium: 118mg

### Ingredients:

- 1 egg; large
- 15 ounces black beans; canned low sodium
- 1 tablespoon of cumin
- 1 tablespoon of smoked paprika
- 1/2 cup of flax meal
- 1 tablespoon of Worcestershire sauce
- 2 tablespoons of onion powder

### Instructions:

Set oven to 400 degrees Fahrenheit. With a fork or potato masher, mash the beans in a large mixing dish. Stir together the egg and Worcestershire sauce in a second, smaller bowl. Add the egg mixture to the beans and combine well. Blend the ingredients well after adding the flax meal &seasonings. Place the dough on a gently oiled cookie sheet lined with parchment paper and shape it into four equal patties. Pat the patties down with a fork until they resemble hamburger patties. Bake each side for 15-20 minutes. Cook until the final temperature is attained; the internal temperature should reach 165 degrees F.

# CHAPTER 5

## Snacks Recipes

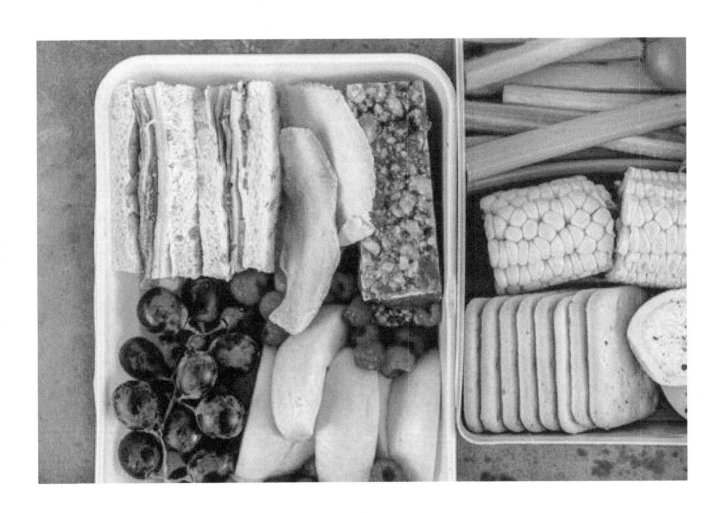

## 61- Almond-Cranberry Celery Logs

Preparation time: 10 minutes

Cooking Time: 0 minutes

Servings: 4

Difficulty Level: Medium

### Nutritional Information:

Calories:72 kcal, protein: 2 g, carbohydrates: 7g, Fat: 4g, Cholesterol: 0mg, Fiber: 1.3g, Sodium:65mg, Potassium:138mg, Phosphorus:33mg, Calcium: 36mg

### Ingredients:

- 4 tbsp mixed berry cream cheese (whipped).
- 4 celery ribs (medium 8-in)
- 12 almonds, dry roasted, whole, unsalted
- 24 dried cranberries: sweetened

### Instructions:

Cut the ends of the celery rib. Fill 1 tablespoon of whipped cream cheese for each celery rib. Break each rib of celery into 3 pieces. Cover each piece with 1 almond and 2 cranberries that have been dried. Cover until ready to eat or refrigerate.

## 62- Asparagus Spread.

Preparation time: 10 minutes

Cooking Time: 0 minutes

Servings: 16

Difficulty Level: Medium

### Nutritional Information:

Calories: 65 kcal, protein: 1g, carbohydrates: 1 g, Fat: 6 g, Cholesterol: 13 mg, Fiber: 0.2 g, Sodium: 56 mg, Potassium: 43 mg, Phosphorus: 18 mg, Calcium: 11 mg

### Ingredients:

- 1/4 cup of mayonnaise
- canned asparagus: 8 ounces (low-sodium)
- 1 tbsp lemon juice
- Cream cheese: 6 ounces
- 2 tbsp onion

### Instructions:

Set out the cream cheese to melt it. Drain asparagus. In a food processor, combine all ingredients and process until blended. Cover it and remove it to refrigerate overnight in a bowl. Serve spread with crackers that are low-sodium or make finger sandwiches.

## 63- German Pancakes

Preparation time: 10 minutes

Cooking Time: 0 minutes

Servings: 10

Difficulty Level: Medium

### Nutritional Information:

Calories:74 kcal, protein:4g, carbohydrates:10g, Fat: 2g, Cholesterol: 76mg, Fiber: 0.2g, Sodium:39mg, Potassium:73mg, Phosphorus:72mg, Calcium: 43 mg

### Ingredients:

- 4 large eggs
- 2 tbsp sugar
- 1/4 tsp vanilla extract
- 1 cup of low-fat milk (1%)
- 2/3 cup of all-purpose flour

### Instructions:

Combine the sugar and flour in a medium dish. Add eggs and mix well with a whisk. Add the vanilla extract and milk and beat smoothly. On a heated 8- or 10-inch non-stick skillet, brush 3 tablespoons of the batter with non-stick cooking spray. Quickly tilt the pan to disperse the batter. Cook until the pancake's underside is brown (about 45 seconds; edges will begin to dry). Cook the other side by flipping the pancake. Continue before it consumes all the batter. Roll thin pancakes to serve with fruit spread, jam, or syrup. Add 1 or 2 teaspoons of ricotta or cream cheese to the filling, if necessary.

## 64   Garlic Oyster Crackers

Preparation time: 10 minutes

Cooking Time: 45- 50 minutes

Servings: 7-8

Difficulty Level: Medium

### Nutritional Information:

Calories:118kcal, protein: 2 g, carbohydrates: 12g, Fat: 7g, Cholesterol: 0 mg, Fiber: 0.3g, Sodium:166mg, Potassium: 21 mg, Phosphorus: 15mg, Calcium: 4mg

### Ingredients:

- 1 tbsp garlic powder
- 1/2 cup of popcorn oil (butter-flavored)
- 2 tsp dried dill weed.
- 7 cups of oyster crackers

### Instructions:

Preheat the oven to 250° F. In a large bowl, mix the oil and garlic powder. Mix the crackers and uniformly coat them. Add the dill weed and toss to combine. Spread on a baking sheet with crackers and bake for 45 minutes. Softly blend after 15 minutes. Scatter crackers on paper towels to cool until ready to serve; store them in an airtight bag.

## 65-   Chicken Pepper Bacon Wraps

Preparation time: 10 minutes

Cooking Time: 10-15 minutes

Servings: 12-24

Difficulty Level: Medium

### Nutritional Information:

Calories:71kcal, protein: 10g, carbohydrates:1g, Fat: 3g, Cholesterol: 26mg, Fiber: 0.8g, Sodium: 96mg, Potassium:147mg, Phosphorus:84mg, Calcium: 9mg

### Ingredients:

- 12 strips of bacon
- 1 onion: medium
- 24 toothpicks (no color dye)
- 12 fresh bananas
- 2 pounds of chicken breast skinless, boneless,
- 12 jalapenos peppers: fresh

### Instructions:

Cut the onion into four pieces. Split bacon into halves. Spray the grill rack using a non-stick cooking spray used for high heat. Pre-heat the outer side of the grill on low or inside of the grill.

Prepare the peppers by removing the seeds from the inside. On one side of the pepper, carve broad ways to break it open. Slice the chicken into at least 24 chunks to fit in the peppers.

Stuff each pepper with one slice of chicken. It is all right if there is any chicken left outside pepper. To cover the chicken, put one slice of the onion on top.

Hold the bacon & wrap it around with toothpicks with onion, chicken, and pepper. To secure them, use multiple toothpicks placed in various directions. Place on the grill. For 10 to 15 minutes, cook bacon until crispy. Turn and flip to avoid burning bacon fire from oil drips.

## 66- Fresh Tofu Spring Rolls

Preparation time: 10 minutes

Cooking Time: 20 minutes

Servings: 6

Difficulty Level: Medium

### Nutritional Information:

Calories:156kcal, protein:8g, carbohydrates:20g, Fat: 5g, Cholesterol: 0mg, Fiber: 1.3g, Sodium:161mg, Potassium:302mg, Phosphorus:93mg, Calcium: 46mg

### Ingredients:

- 2 carrots: medium
- 12 leaves: Romaine lettuce
- 1/2 red onion: medium
- 1/4 tsp of sea salt
- 1/2 tbsp ground cumin
- Firm tofu: 16 ounces
- For spring rolls:12 rice wrappers
- 1/2 tbsp garlic: granulated
- 1 tbsp of olive oil
- 1/2 tsp black pepper

### Instructions:

Clean the lettuce, dry it, and split each leaf in half lengthwise. Cut Onion and Carrots in Julienne Type. Boil 6 cups of water and later set aside for the rice wrappers to soak. Drain and cover the tofu to dry. Split it into 12 pieces, each roughly 4 inches long. Spread the tofu on a plate with granulated garlic, cumin, black pepper, and sea salt and season it uniformly.

Heat olive oil in a non-stick skillet. Put the tofu strips down the seasoned side in the pan. Season the other side and fry for around 1 or 2 minutes until the base is lightly browned. Turn the other side and fry until lightly browned. To cool, place the tofu on a tray.

In a wide, deep bowl, pour hot water. Drop a rice wrapper in hot water. Until it is slightly soft, put the wrapper on a large plate and put two halves of the lettuce in the wrapper's middle. Scatter on top of the lettuce with 2 to 3 tablespoons of carrot and 1 to 2 tablespoons of sliced onion. On top of the vegetables, place one cooled tofu strip. Fold the sides in and then firmly fold the bottom up and roll. Repeat for the rest of the strips of tofu, rice wrappers, and vegetables. With your preferred low-sodium sauce, serve it.

## 67-Santa Fe French Toast

Preparation time: 10 minutes

Cooking Time: 10 minutes

Servings: 4

Difficulty Level: Medium

### Nutritional Information:

Calories: 218 kcal, protein: 10 g, carbohydrates: 13 g, Fat: 14 g, Cholesterol: 186 mg, Fiber: 2.0 g, Sodium: 241 mg, Potassium: 193 mg, Phosphorus: 165 mg, Calcium: 167 mg

### Ingredients:

- 4 eggs
- 4 slices of white bread, 3/4" thick
- 2 tablespoons of canola oil
- 1-1/4 cup of almond milk: unsweetened

### Instructions:

Preheat the oven to 400º F. Cut the crust and slice the bread in half diagonally. Add to the almond milk slightly beaten eggs. Pour oil into a pan and heat it. Dip the bread into a mixture of eggs. Fry in oil until all sides are brown. Place pieces of browned toast on a hot baking dish. In the oven, cook for 4 minutes to puff up the toast. Remove from the oven and, if possible, drain on paper towels. Serve with syrup jelly or powdered sugar.

# 68- Baked Shrimp Rolls

Preparation time: 10 minutes

Cooking Time: 30-40 minutes

Servings: 6

Difficulty Level: Medium

## Nutritional Information:

Calories:208kcal, protein: 16g, carbohydrates:30g, Fat: 2g, Cholesterol: 91mg, Fiber: 1.5g, Sodium:292mg, Potassium: 255mg, Phosphorus: 166 mg, Calcium: 65mg

## Ingredients:

- 1/2 cup of carrots
- 2 cups of Napa cabbage
- 1/4 cup of green onions
- 12 egg roll wrappers: 7" square
- 1 tsp ginger root
- 2 tbsp fresh cilantro
- 1 tbsp of hoisin sauce
- 1-1/2 cups of raw shrimp
- 1 tsp of brown sugar
- 1/4 tsp red chili flakes (optional)
- 1 tsp garlic powder
- 3 tbsp water

## Instructions:

Preheat the oven to 400° F. If it is frozen, set the egg roll wrappers out to defrost them. Shred the carrots and cabbage finely. Slice the onions thinly and chop the cilantro. Grate the Ginger. Wash and cut the shrimp finely. Add carrots, cabbage, green onions, and shrimp to a non-stick pre-heated skillet.

Stir fry until the shrimp and vegetables are pink, translucent, and tender; stir periodically (about 8 minutes). Add hoisin sauce, cilantro, garlic powder, brown sugar, red chili flakes, and ginger. Mix properly so the spices are equally

distributed. Cook for another 2 minutes, then remove from the heat and drain the excess oil.

Spray canola oil on a baking sheet while the veggie shrimp mixture is cooling; put it aside. On the cutting board (or any other clean surfaces), arrange spring roll wrappers and fill as follows: Put one spoonful tablespoon of cooked mixture in each, diagonally, around one-third from the top of the wrapper, not directly in the center. Fold two opposite wrapper edges over the filling and roll first on the shorter side and then on the longer side until it's done.

Dip a finger into the water and rub to close the edge of the finished roll, and put the edge's folded side on the baking sheet. Use a canola oil spray to spray each loaded spring roll. Bake for about 20 minutes; turn after 10 minutes. Rolls should be crispy and finely browned.

# 69- Fiesta Roll-Ups

Preparation time: 10 minutes

Cooking Time: 0 minutes

Servings: 8-12

Difficulty Level: Medium

## Nutritional Information:

Calories: 148 kcal, protein: 3 g, carbohydrates: 16 g, Fat: 8 g, Cholesterol: 21 mg, Fiber: 0.9 g, Sodium: 260 mg, Potassium: 73 mg, Phosphorus: 52 mg, Calcium: 39 mg

## Ingredients:

- 1/2 tsp cumin
- 1/2 tsp garlic powder
- 4 tbsp green onion
- 1/2 tsp of chili powder
- 6 flour tortillas:8" size
- 8 ounces of cream cheese
- 4 ounces of chopped green chilies: canned.

## Instructions:

Set out the cream cheese to melt it. Slice the green onions thinly. Combine the spices, green onions, and green chili in a dish. Mix with the softened cream cheese. Place a small amount of cream cheese mixture on each tortilla, leaving 1/4" of the edge exposed. Roll out the tortillas like a roll of jelly. To hold the rolls, use a toothpick. Cover for at least one hour and refrigerate. Cut into 1-inch pieces and serve as an appetizer or snack.

## 70- Corn and Cheese Balls

Preparation time: 10 minutes

Cooking Time: 20 minutes

Servings: 4-5

Difficulty Level: Medium

### Nutritional Information:

Calories: 253 kcal, protein: 7 g, carbohydrates: 27 g, Fat: 13 g, Cholesterol: 3 mg, Fiber: 2.3 g, Sodium: 287 mg, Potassium: 169 mg, Phosphorus: 86 mg, Calcium: 46 mg

### Ingredients:

- 1 green chili
- 2 cups of yellow Corn: frozen
- 2 tbsp cilantro
- 4 slices of White Bread
- 2 cups of vegetable oil
- 1/2 cup of cottage cheese
- 1 tsp chili powder
- 1/2 cup of all-purpose white flour
- 1 tsp of cumin powder
- 1/4 tsp of salt
- 1 tsp of cilantro powder

### Instructions:

Boil Corn and finely chop the cilantro and green chili. Blend the cheese and thawed Corn in a

mixing pot. Soak the slices of bread in water, then squeeze the water out so that the bread is dry. Add this to the combination of Corn and cheese. Add flour, cilantro, and dried spices. Gently blend it. In a big saucepan, heat the oil. Shape small balls of the cheese and corn mixture using a tablespoon and drop each ball into the hot oil. Cook until brown and golden.

Take out the balls and put them on a kitchen napkin tray to drain the excess oil. Serve hot with Cilantro Chutney.

## 71-Cottage Cheese Pancakes with Fresh Strawberries

Preparation time: 10 minutes

Cooking Time: 20 minutes

Servings: 6

Difficulty Level: Medium

### Nutritional Information:

Calories: 253 kcal, protein: 11 g, carbohydrates: 21 g, Fat: 17 g, Cholesterol: 182 mg, Fiber: 2.0 g, Sodium: 172 mg, Potassium: 217 mg, Phosphorus: 159 mg, Calcium: 64 mg

### Ingredients:

- 1/2 cup of white flour: all-purpose
- Lightly beat 4 large eggs.
- 3 cups of strawberries, sliced. (fresh)
- 6 tbsp melted butter: unsalted.
- 1 cup of cottage cheese

### Instructions:

Combine the eggs (lightly beaten), cottage cheese, melted butter, and flour in a medium-sized dish. Spray with non-stick cooking spray or butter on the grill or frying pan. Over medium to high heat, warm the griddle or frying pan. Ladle around 1/4 cup of batter to shape pancakes on the griddle (about 4" in diameter). Cook the pancakes until the undersides are gently browned for 2-3 minutes, then change the other side to brown.

Move the pancakes to a platter that is heated. Continue with the leftover batter to create pancakes. With 1/2 cup sliced strawberries, top each serving of pancakes.

## 72-Veggie Pizza Snacks

Preparation time: 10 minutes

Cooking Time: 20 minutes

Servings: 10-12

Difficulty Level: Medium

### Nutritional Information:

Calories: 90 kcal, protein: 2 g, carbohydrates: 7 g, Fat: 6 g, Cholesterol: 11 mg, Fiber: 0.4 g, Sodium: 135 mg, Potassium: 76 mg, Phosphorus: 37 mg, Calcium: 18 mg

### Ingredients:

- 2 tbsp ranch salad dressing: low-fat
- 1/2 cup of sour cream
- 1/4 tsp garlic powder
- Crescent roll dough: 16 ounces
- 1 cup of cream cheese: whipped.
- 1 carrot: medium
- 1 cup of broccoli florets
- 1/2 cucumber: medium
- 1/2 cup of cherry tomatoes
- 1/2 cup of red onion

### Instructions:

Spray a baking pan of 13" x 9" x 2" with non-stick cooking spray and ready the oven by preheating it to 350º F. Into the baking tray, spread out packs of crescent rolls, turning into a single smooth dough surface. Bake for 10 to 15 minutes. Let it rest for 10 to 15 minutes before it cools off. Beat the sour cream and cream cheese

in a bowl until it is smooth. Stir in the garlic powder and ranch dressing. Layer the paste over the crust equally. Chop the broccoli, carrot, onion, and cucumber. Cut the cherry tomatoes into slices. Arrange the sliced vegetables on top of the mixture of cream cheese. Cover and refrigerate the pizza with plastic wrap before serving time.

## 73-Flour Tortilla Chips

Preparation time: 5 minutes

Cooking Time: 10 minutes

Servings: 6

Difficulty Level: Easy

### Nutritional Information:

Calories: 163 kcal, protein: 2 g, carbohydrates: 14 g, Fat: 11 g, Cholesterol: 0 mg, Fiber: 0.7 g, Sodium: 292 mg, Potassium: 41 mg, Phosphorus: 54 mg, Calcium: 36 mg

### Ingredients:

- 1/2 cup of canola oil
- 6 flour tortillas:6" size

### Instructions:

Slice each tortilla into 8 wedge-shaped bits. In a heavy skillet, heat the sufficient oil to cover ¼ inch of the skillet. Add the tortilla pieces while the oil is hot and turn once light golden and crispy. On paper towels, drop the chips and drain them. Store the chips in sealed bags until they are fit for consumption.

## 74-Cereal Snack Mix with Salt-free Seasoning

Preparation time: 20 minutes

Cooking Time: 60 minutes

Servings: 12

Difficulty Level: Easy

## Nutritional Information:

Calories: 195 kcal, protein: 3 g, carbohydrates: 30 g, Fat: 7 g, Cholesterol: 15 mg, Fiber: 1.0 g, Sodium: 157 mg, Potassium: 124 mg, Phosphorus: 38 mg, Calcium: 16 mg

## Ingredients:

- 8 cups of cereal
- 3 tbsp Herb and Onion seasoning blend
- 2 cups of oyster crackers
- 6 tbsp of butter: unsalted
- 2 cups of pretzels: unsalted

## Instructions:

Preheat the oven to 250° F. In a small baking tray, heat the butter. Stir in spices. Toss in the cereal, oyster crackers, pretzels, and cover with the butter mixture. Cook for 60 minutes, remove the pan from the oven and stir after 15 minutes.

## 75- Chicken Nuggets with Honey Mustard Dipping Sauce

Preparation time: 10 minutes

Cooking Time: 20 minutes

Servings: 12

Difficulty Level: Medium

## Nutritional Information:

Calories: 164 kcal, protein: 9 g, carbohydrates: 14 g, Fat: 8 g, Cholesterol: 25 mg, Fiber: 0.3 g, Sodium: 157 mg, Potassium: 99 mg, Phosphorus: 70 mg, Calcium: 11 mg

## Ingredients:

- 1/2 cup of mayonnaise
- 1 tbsp yellow mustard
- 2 tsp Worcestershire sauce

- 1/3 cup of honey
- 2 tbsp 1% low-fat milk
- 1 large egg
- 1-pound chicken breast: boneless
- 3 cups of cornflakes

## Instructions:

In a small bowl, stir the mayonnaise, mustard, Worcestershire sauce, and honey together. Cool the sauce before the nuggets are fried to serve as a dipping sauce.

Preheat the oven to 400° F. Cut 36 bite-sized chicken breast pieces. Crush the cornflakes and drop the crumbs into a wide bag with a Ziplock. Mix the beaten egg & milk in a small bowl. Dip the chicken pieces in the egg mixture, then shake it to cover with cornflake crumbs in a zip-lock container. Bake the nuggets for 15 minutes or until finished on a baking sheet coated with non-stick cooking spray.

## 76-Cranberry Cabbage

Preparation time: 5 minutes

Cooking Time: 10 minutes

Servings: 8

Difficulty Level: Easy

## Nutritional Information:

Calories: 73 kcal, protein: 1 g, carbohydrates: 18 g, Fat: 0 g, Cholesterol: 0 mg, Fiber: 1.6 g, Sodium: 32 mg, Potassium: 138 mg, Phosphorus: 18 mg, Calcium: 25 mg

## Ingredients:

- 1 medium red cabbage
- canned whole-berry cranberry sauce: 10 ounces
- 1/4 tsp ground cloves
- 1 tbsp of fresh lemon juice

## Instructions:

Heat the cloves, cranberry sauce, and lemon juice in a large pan and bring them to a boil. Add the cabbage to the melted cranberry sauce and mix well. Bring the mixture to a boil; reduce heat. Continue to cook until the cabbage is soft; keep stirring. Serve it warm.

## 77-Chicken Parmesan Meatballs

Preparation time: 10 minutes

Cooking Time: 30 minutes

Servings: 10

Difficulty Level: Medium

## Nutritional Information:

Calories: 114 kcal, protein: 11 g, carbohydrates: 4 g, Fat: 6 g, Cholesterol: 64 mg, Fiber: 0.5 g, Sodium: 223 mg, Potassium: 350 mg, Phosphorus: 132 mg, Calcium: 59 mg

## Ingredients:

- 3 tbsp breadcrumbs
- 1 large egg
- ground chicken: 1 pound
- 1 tbsp Parmesan cheese: grated.
- 1/4 tsp Italian seasoning
- pizza sauce: 8 ounces
- 1/4 tsp onion powder
- 1/2 cup of mozzarella cheese: shredded
- 1/4 tsp garlic powder

## Instructions:

Spray with cooking spray on a large baking dish and pre-heat the oven to 375 ° F. Mix egg, ground chicken, parmesan cheese, breadcrumbs, spices, and 2 teaspoons of pizza sauce in a bowl. Shape 30 small meatballs around the size of a ping-pong ball; put meatballs on the baking sheet that has been prepared. For 15 minutes, bake them.

Spread the bottom of a glass baking dish with a thin coat of pizza sauce. In a glass baking dish, put the meatballs. Then add shredded mozzarella to the leftover pizza sauce on top of the meatballs. Put it back in the oven and cook for an extra 10 minutes.

## 78- Seafood Dip

Preparation time: 15 minutes

Cooking Time: 0 minutes

Servings: 10

Difficulty Level: Easy

## Nutritional Information:

Calories: 187 kcal, protein: 8 g, carbohydrates: 14 g, Fat: 11 g, Cholesterol: 71 mg, Fiber: 0.2 g, Sodium: 256 mg, Potassium: 163 mg, Phosphorus: 82 mg, Calcium: 50 mg

## Ingredients:

- 4 ounces imitation crabmeat
- 8 ounces cooked shrimp
- 1 cup ketchup: no salt.
- Cream cheese: 8 ounces
- 1 tbsp lemon juice
- 1-1/2 tbsp prepared horseradish
- 1 tbsp low-sodium Worcestershire sauce.
- 30 crackers: low-sodium
- 1/2 tsp hot sauce

## Instructions:

To melt the cream cheese, remove it from the refrigerator, do not use the oven. According to package instructions, thaw shrimp. Remove the shrimp shells and any visible veins and break them into tiny parts.

Chop the crab meat imitation into smaller fragments. Stir together the shrimp and crab meat and put them in the refrigerator. To produce a low-sodium cocktail sauce, mix horseradish, ketchup, Worcestershire sauce, and lemon juice in a small bowl. Stir the softened cream cheese in a medium bowl until it becomes smooth. To the cream cheese, steadily add the cocktail sauce. Thoroughly stir.

Then add a small amount of hot sauce. Thoroughly stir. Sample the mixture of cream cheese. If required, add more sauce. Add the crabmeat and shrimp to the cream cheese. Thoroughly stir. Check the mixture of cream cheese. If required, add more sauce. Cover and cool overnight in the refrigerator. Serve with low-sodium crackers.

## 79- Buffalo Wings

Preparation time: 10 minutes

Cooking Time: 40 minutes

Servings: 12

Difficulty Level: Medium

### Nutritional Information:

Calories: 131 kcal, protein: 8 g, carbohydrates: 0 g, Fat: 11 g, Cholesterol: 63 mg, Fiber: 0g, Sodium: 64 mg, Potassium: 105 mg, Phosphorus: 61 mg, Calcium: 8 mg

### Ingredients:

- 1/3 cup of hot pepper sauce
- 8 tbsp butter: unsalted
- 1/4 cup of tomato sauce: low-sodium
- 1/4 cup of roasted red pepper sauce.
- 1/2 tsp garlic powder
- 1 tbsp olive oil
- 24 chicken wing drumettes
- 1/2 tsp Italian seasoning blend: dried

### Instructions:

Preheat the oven to 400° F. In a saucepan, heat the sugar. Combine and stir in the red pepper sauce, spicy sauce, olive oil, tomato sauce, Italian seasonings, and garlic powder. Remove the pan from heat. In a baking dish, put the

chicken wings. Over the wings, pour the sauce and bake for 30 to 35 minutes. When ready to eat, serve the wings hot or put them in a heated warming dish or crockpot.

## 80- Buffalo Chicken Dip

Preparation time: 10 minutes

Cooking Time: 30 minutes

Servings: 16

Difficulty Level: Medium

### Nutritional Information:

Calories: 86 kcal, protein: 6 g, carbohydrates: 2 g, Fat: 6 g, Cholesterol: 29 mg, Fiber: 0 g, Sodium: 109 mg, Potassium: 89 mg, Phosphorus: 56 mg, Calcium: 26 mg

### Ingredients:

- 1 cup of low-fat sour cream.
- 4 ounces softened cream cheese.
- 4 tsp of hot pepper sauce
- ½ tsp of garlic powder (optional)
- 2 cups of chicken: cooked and shredded

### Instructions:

Mix the cream cheese and the sour cream in a medium bowl until smooth. Add 2 teaspoons of sauce and stir it. Add the chicken and blend softly. Add 1⁄2 teaspoon of additional hot sauce at a time; sample and proceed to add more hot sauce to the level you like.

Put the mixture over low heat in a slow cooker for 2 to 3 hours, or bake in the oven for 30 minutes at 350 °F. For dipping, serve a warm dip with broccoli, cauliflower, tortilla chips, cucumber, and celery.

## 81- Avocado Dip

Preparation time: 10 minutes

Cooking Time: 0 minutes

Servings: 8

Difficulty Level: Easy

## Nutritional Information:

Calories: 64 kcal, protein: 1 g, carbohydrates: 4 g, Fat: 6 g, Cholesterol: 1 mg, Fiber: 2 g, Sodium: 77 mg, Potassium: 140 mg, Phosphorus: 4 mg, Calcium: 27 mg

## Ingredients:

- 1/2 ripe avocado
- 2 oz of cream cheese
- 1/2 tsp. of sugar
- 1 lime
- 1/8 tsp. of ground pepper
- 1/8 tsp. of salt

## Instructions:

Soften the cream cheese at room temperature. Halve the avocado and cut the kernel. Scoop the fruit from the avocado using a spoon, leaving the skin. Mix the cream cheese and the avocado in a food processor or blender. Squeeze the limes and add the juice to the mixer. Stir in the butter, salt, and pepper and combine until smooth.

## 82- Crunchy Crunch

Preparation time: 10 minutes

Cooking Time: 60 minutes

Servings: 12

Difficulty Level: Easy

## Nutritional Information:

Calories: 92 kcal, protein: 1 g, carbohydrates: 14 g, Fat: 3 g, Cholesterol: 0 mg, Fiber: 0.4 g, Sodium: 127 mg, Potassium: 37 mg, Phosphorus: 16 mg, Calcium: 3 mg

## Ingredients:

- 2 cups of white bread in cubes
- 4 cups of Cheerios
- 1/2 tsp of garlic powder
- 1/4 cup of margarine, melted.
- 1/4 tsp of black pepper
- 4 cups of Shredded Wheat Minis
- 1/2 cup of oil
- 1 tsp of onion powder

## Instructions:

Preheat the oven to 250 degrees F. Mix the bread cubes and cereal in a large bowl. Melt the margarine in a shallow bowl. Add margarine over a mixture of cereal. Add the oil, onion powder, garlic powder, and black pepper to taste in a cereal mixture. Always stir properly. Spread the mixture over 2 sheets of cookies. For 1 hour, bake it. Cool and place in a jar that is covered.

## 83- Grilled Salsa

Preparation time: 5 minutes

Cooking Time: 10 minutes

Servings: 8

Difficulty Level: Easy

## Nutritional Information:

Calories: 14 kcal, protein: 1 g, carbohydrates: 2 g, Fat: 1 g, Cholesterol: 0 mg, Fiber: 0 g, Sodium: 4 mg, Potassium: 117 mg, Phosphorus: 14 mg, Calcium: 10 mg

## Ingredients:

- 2 large onions (cut in 3 rings)
- 2 lbs. tomatillos
- 4 garlic cloves: large
- 2 lbs. Roma tomatoes
- 6 serrano chilies
- 1 bag of small peppers (orange, yellow, red) or large ones

- 1 bunch of cilantro leaves
- 6 Tbsp of lemon or lime juice
- 2 tsp of salt

## Instructions:

On the grill, roast the tomatoes, chilies, onions, and peppers until mildly blackened, or grill until barely blackened. In the blender or food processor, place small amounts of each vegetable. Finely chopped up. Mix well and add minced cilantro, garlic, lemon/lime juice, and spice. Refrigerate. For milder salsa, reduce the number of Serrano chilies.

## 84    Craisin Slice

Preparation time: 10 minutes

Cooking Time: 40 minutes

Servings: 12

Difficulty Level: Medium

## Nutritional Information:

Calories: 136 kcal, protein: 1 g, carbohydrates: 15 g, Fat: 8 g, Cholesterol: 29 mg, Fiber: 0 g, Sodium: 157 mg, Potassium: 99 mg, Phosphorus: 70 mg, Calcium: 11 mg

## Ingredients:

- 1 cup of caster sugar
- 300g margarine: unsalted
- 2 ½ cups of plain flour
- One egg white (lightly beaten).
- 125g craisins (dried cranberries)
- 2 tbsp of caster sugar, extra
- Cinnamon, pinch

## Instructions:

Preheat the oven to 300 degrees Fahrenheit. Line and grease a Swiss roll tray that is 26cm ×32cm. Add the margarine, caster sugar, and flour into a food processor. Mix it until smooth. Often, this may be done by hand. Use the raisins and cinnamon to stir. The mixture is then transferred onto the prepared tray. Brush with white eggs and sprinkle the extra caster sugar on it. For about 40 minutes, bake it in the oven or until brown. Cool it and split it into finger-sized pieces.

## 85-   Garlic bread

Preparation time: 10 minutes

Cooking Time: 10 minutes

Servings: 16 slices

Difficulty Level: Medium

## Nutritional Information:

Calories: 76 kcal, protein: 3 g, carbohydrates: 16 g, Fat: 0 g, Cholesterol: 0 mg, Fiber: 0.6 g, Sodium: 55 mg, Potassium: 25 mg, Phosphorus: 26 mg, Calcium: 5 mg

## Ingredients:

- 1 x 170g of French breadstick (about 25cm long)
- 2 tbsp low salt margarine
- 3 tsp crushed garlic
- 2 tsp skim milk
- 1 tbsp chopped parsley

## Instructions:

Heat the margarine for one minute in a small mixing dish. Slowly pour in the milk, around half a teaspoon at a time. Toss in the parsley and garlic, and blend properly. Cut a stick of bread into 16 slices. Brush margarine over the top of every slice. On a flat tray, place the bread slices under the griller until the bread is lightly browned.

## 86-   Fried Onion Rings

Preparation time: 5 minutes

Cooking Time: 10 minutes

Servings: 8

Difficulty Level: Easy

## Nutritional Information:

Calories: 175 kcal, protein: 2.1 g, carbohydrates: 20 g, Fat: 9.9 g, Cholesterol: 16 mg, Fiber: 1.3 g, Sodium: 288 mg, Potassium: 76 mg, Phosphorus: 13.9 mg, Calcium: 36 mg

## Ingredients:

- ¼ cup flour: all-purpose
- ¾ cup of plain cornmeal
- 1 tsp sugar
- ½ cup of vegetable oil for frying
- 1 beaten egg.
- 4 onions: medium
- ¼ cup of water

## Instructions:

Mix the flour, sugar, and cornmeal; set aside. Peel the onions and split them approximately 1/4" thick crosswise. Divide them into circles. The beaten egg and water are combined. In egg wash, dip circles, then coat cornmeal mixture. Fry onion rings in hot vegetable oil for 3-5 minutes, turning until brown. On a paper towel, rinse. Serve hot.

## 87- Coconut Rainbow Marshmallows

Preparation time: 10 minutes

Cooking Time: 20 minutes

Servings: 12

Difficulty Level: Medium

## Nutritional Information:

Calories: 164 kcal, protein: 9 g, carbohydrates: 14 g, Fat: 8 g, Cholesterol: 25 mg, Fiber: 0.3 g, Sodium: 157 mg, Potassium: 99 mg, Phosphorus: 70 mg, Calcium: 11 mg

## Ingredients:

- 1 cup of cold water
- 4 tbsp gelatin
- 2 cups of hot water
- 4 cups of caster sugar

**Flavoring and food color (use one combination)**

- Peppermint:1/2 tsp of peppermint essence and 6 drops of green food coloring
- Orange:1 tsp orange blossom water and ½ tsp orange food coloring
- Rose: 1 tsp rosewater and ¼ tsp of rose or red food coloring
- 1 cup coconut: desiccated
- 2 tsp lemon juice

## Instructions:

Add a cup of the gelatin to cool water. In a wide saucepan, mix the sugar and hot water; whisk over low heat until the sugar dissolves; bring it to a simmer. Add gelatin mixture; cook continuously for 20 minutes, uncovered from cool to lukewarm. In an electric mixer, pour the sugar mixture and add lemon juice, coloring, and flavoring. Beat at high speed until the mixture is thick and keeps its form for around 5 minutes. Rinse the 20x30 pan with cold water; do not dry. Spread the pan with the marshmallow mixture. Sprinkle over the marshmallow mixture with a little coconut. Allow setting at room temperature for about 2 hours until firm. Slice the marshmallow, using a wet knife, into 40 squares (about 4x4cm each). Toss in the remaining coconut.

## 88- Homemade Yeast Rolls

Preparation time: 10-20 minutes

Cooking Time: 20 minutes

Servings: 10-15

Difficulty Level: Medium

## Nutritional Information:

Calories: 148 kcal, protein: 3 g, carbohydrates: 24 g, Fat: 4 g, Cholesterol: 6 mg, Fiber: 0.2 g, Sodium: 5 mg, Potassium: 31 mg, Phosphorus: 32 mg, Calcium: 5 mg

## Ingredients:

- 1/4 cup of sugar
- 3 1/2 cup of all-purpose flour
- 1/4 cup of margarine or butter soften.
- 1/2 cup of warm water (120 to 130°F)
- quick-acting dry yeast: 1 package
- 1 large egg
- 1/2 cup of warm skim milk (cooled to 120 to 130°F)

## Instructions:

In a 2 1/2-quart bowl, mix 2 cups of sugar, flour, yeast, and margarine. Add skim milk, egg, and water. Beat for 1 minute at a low mixer level, scraping the bowl. Stir in the leftover flour to make it easy to handle the dough. Place the dough onto a lightly floured surface; knead for approximately 5 minutes until smooth and elastic.

Put in a 2- 1/2-quart greased bowl. Cover and let it rise until the dough doubles in size, for around 1 hour, in a warm place. If the indentation persists when touched, the dough is ready. Punch down dough. Roll or split into desired shapes. Brush the butter or margarine. Cover and let it rise until the size doubles for around thirty minutes. Preheat the oven to 400 degrees F. Bake for 12 to 18 minutes, until golden brown.

## 89-  Baked eggplant fries

Preparation time: 10 minutes

Cooking Time: 30 minutes

Servings: 6

Difficulty Level: Easy

## Nutritional Information:

Calories: 233 kcal, protein: 5 g, carbohydrates: 25 g, Fat: 12 g, Cholesterol: 47 mg, Fiber: 2 g, Sodium: 211 mg, Potassium: 214 mg, Phosphorus: 85 mg, Calcium: 60 mg

## Ingredients:

- ½ tsp garlic powder
- 2 eggs
- 1 eggplant: medium, peeled, and slashed into fries.
- ½ tsp of dried oregano
- 1 1/2 cups of cornmeal
- 1 tbsp olive oil
- ½ tsp paprika

## Instructions:

Preheat the oven to 400 degrees F. Grease the baking sheet slightly. In a medium dish, combine the oregano, paprika, cornmeal, and garlic powder. In a cup, break two eggs and beat them gently. Coat the eggplant fries with beaten eggs and cornmeal mixture. On a baking sheet, put the eggplant fries and bake for 20-25 minutes, flipping them after 12 minutes.

## 90-  Baked Pita Chips

Preparation time: 5 minutes

Cooking Time: 15 minutes

Servings: 6

Difficulty Level: Easy

## Nutritional Information:

Calories: 137 kcal, protein: 2.5 g, carbohydrates: 15.4 g, Fat: 7 g, Cholesterol: 0 mg, Fiber: 0.6 g, Sodium: 148 mg, Potassium: 33 mg, Phosphorus: 27 mg, Calcium: 106 mg

## Ingredients:

- Chili powder to taste.
- 3 Tbsp. of olive oil
- 3 (6") pita rounds

## Instructions:

Split the pitas using kitchen scissors into 2 rounds. Cut each into 8 wedges. Brush the olive oil on pita wedges and dust with the chili powder. Bake for about 15 minutes at 350 °F or until crisp.

## 91-  Grilled Herb Corn

Preparation time: 5 minutes

Cooking Time: 10-15 minutes

Servings: 8

Difficulty Level: Easy

## Nutritional Information:

Calories: 183 kcal, protein: 3 g, carbohydrates: 18 g, Fat: 13 g, Cholesterol: 31 mg, Fiber: 2 g, Sodium: 106 mg, Potassium: 237 mg, Phosphorus: 63 mg, Calcium: 13 mg

## Ingredients:

- 2 tbsp of parsley, minced.
- 1–2 fresh limes
- 1/2 cup of butter, unsalted
- 2 tbsp of fresh chives, minced.
- 1/2 tsp of cayenne pepper (or per taste)
- 1 tsp of dried thyme
- 8 ears of sweet corn (husked).

## Instructions:

Beat the butter, parsley, chives, thyme, and cayenne pepper in a small bowl until combined. Spread a mixture of 1 tablespoon over each ear of corn. Individually, cover Corn in heavy-duty foil. Grill the Corn, coated, for 10-15 minutes over medium heat or until soft, rotating

periodically. To make steam escape, open the foil carefully.

## 92-  Crispy Tortilla Pizza

Preparation time: 10 minutes

Cooking Time: 20-25 minutes

Servings: 2

Difficulty Level: Medium

## Nutritional Information:

Calories: 326 kcal, protein: 15 g, carbohydrates: 35 g, Fat: 14 g, Cholesterol: 61 mg, Fiber: 2.4 g, Sodium: 572 mg, Potassium: 397 mg, Phosphorus: 194 mg, Calcium: 75 mg

## Ingredients:

- Butter or substitute
- 4 tbsp marinara sauce
- cream cheese: 2 ounces
- 1/4 cup of broccoli
- 2 flour tortillas: 8-inch size
- 1/4 cup of red onion
- 2 ounces of grilled chicken
- 1/4 cup of fresh mushrooms

## Instructions:

Preheat the oven to 400º F. Set out cream cheese to melt it. Cut and slice broccoli, mushrooms, and onion finely. Brush both sides of each flour tortilla with butter spray and arrange on a baking tray lined with aluminum foil. In the oven, bake tortillas until golden brown; turn them after 5 to 10 minutes as required. Take out the tortillas from the oven, cover each with 1-ounce cream cheese, and layer with 2 teaspoons of marinara sauce. Strip the chicken, put 1 ounce of chicken on each tortilla, and cover it with vegetables. Cook it in the oven for 5 minutes at 400º F until the vegetables get soft. Takeout from the oven, split it into quarters, and enjoy it.

## 93- Sugar and Spice Popcorn

Preparation time: 5 minutes

Cooking Time: 5 minutes

Servings: 4

Difficulty Level: Easy

### Nutritional Information:

Calories: 120 kcal, protein: 2 g, carbohydrates: 12 g, Fat: 7 g, Cholesterol: 16 mg, Fiber: 2.5g, Sodium: 2 mg, Potassium: 56 mg, Phosphorus: 60 mg, Calcium: 6 mg

### Ingredients:

- 2 tbsp of unsalted butter
- 8 cups of air-popped popcorn
- 2 tbsp of sugar
- 1/4 tsp of nutmeg
- 1/2 tsp of cinnamon

### Instructions:

Puff popcorn; put it aside. In the microwave or a saucepan on the burner, heat the cinnamon, sugar, butter, and nutmeg until the butter melts and sugar dissolves; do not burn the butter. Drizzle the popcorn with the spiced butter mixture, and blend properly. For best results, serve instantly.

## 94  Cornmeal Cookies

Preparation time: 10 minutes

Cooking Time: 20 minutes

Servings: 24

Difficulty Level: Easy

### Nutritional Information:

Calories: 156 kcal, protein: 2 g, carbohydrates: 19 g, Fat: 8 g, Cholesterol: 22 mg, Fiber: 0.6 g,

Sodium: 52 mg, Potassium: 25 mg, Phosphorus: 23 mg, Calcium: 23 mg

### Ingredients:

- 1-1/2 cups of white flour: all-purpose
- 1 cup of yellow cornmeal: finely ground.
- 1-1/2 tsp of baking powder.
- 1 cup of unsalted butter (2 sticks)
- 1/8 tsp of salt
- 1 cup of granulated sugar
- 1 tsp vanilla extract
- 1/2 cup of liquid egg substitute: low cholesterol

### Instructions:

Preheat the oven to 350° F. Grease the tray for baking. Sift the flour, cornmeal, salt, and baking powder in a mixing bowl. Put aside. Cream the butter and the sugar in a separate mixing bowl until light and fluffy. Beat in vanilla extract substitute and an egg. Stir in the butter mixture with the dry ingredients and beat until well mixed. Add spoonful teaspoons of the mixture in rows about 2" apart onto the greased baking sheet. Bake until the cookies are golden brown from the outside for 7 to 8 minutes. To cool, shift to a wire rack.

## 95-  Almond Meringue Cookies

Preparation time: 10 minutes

Cooking Time: 30 minutes

Servings: 6

Difficulty Level: Medium

### Nutritional Information:

Calories: 37.9 kcal, protein: 0.6 g, carbohydrates: 9 g, Fat: 0 g, Cholesterol: 0 mg, Fiber: 0 g, Sodium: 18 mg, Potassium: 51 mg, Phosphorus: 0.85 mg, Calcium: 1 mg

## Ingredients:

- ½ cup of white sugar
- 2 egg whites
- ½ tsp of almond extract
- 1 tsp of cream of tartar
- ½ tsp of vanilla extract

## Instructions:

Preheat the oven to 300°F.Beat the egg whites with tartar cream until the amount has doubled. Add the rest of the ingredients and beat until they form strong peaks. Layer one tsp full of meringue with the spoon's help onto a parchment-lined baking sheet using two teaspoons. Bake for around 25 minutes at 300°F or until the mixture is crisp. Store in an airtight jar.

## 96- Mug Meat Loaf

Preparation time: 5 minutes

Cooking Time: 15 minutes

Servings: 2

Difficulty Level: Medium

## Nutritional Information:

Calories: 205 kcal, protein: 17 g, carbohydrates: 14 g, Fat: 9 g, Cholesterol: 81 mg, Fiber: 0.4 g, Sodium: 263 mg, Potassium: 254mg, Phosphorus: 147 mg, Calcium: 36 mg

## Ingredients:

- 1/4-pound of lean ground beef
- 2 tbsp quick-cooking oats
- 2 tbsp 1% low-fat milk
- 1 tsp onion powder
- 2 tsp ketchup

## Instructions:

Use cooking spray to coat a 12-ounce microwave-safe bowl. Mix the onion powder,

milk (or replacer), ketchup, and oats in a cup. Blend beef and paste properly and pat in a cup. Microwave it covered for 3 minutes or until the meat is cooked.

## 97- Corn Idlis

Preparation time: 10 minutes

Cooking Time: 20 minutes

Servings: 4

Difficulty Level: Medium

## Nutritional Information:

Calories: 175 kcal, protein: 5 g, carbohydrates: 14 g, Fat: 11 g, Cholesterol: 4 mg, Fiber: 0.8 g, Sodium: 214 mg, Potassium: 140 mg, Phosphorus: 89 mg, Calcium: 69 mg

## Ingredients:

- 1 tsp mustard seeds
- 2 tbsp vegetable oil
- 1/4 cup of semolina
- 1/8 tsp salt
- 2 green chilies are finely chopped.
- 1/4 cup of yogurt
- 1 tbsp ghee (clarified butter)
- 1/4 cup of Corn, grated.
- 1 tbsp chopped cilantro finely.
- 1/4 cup of water
- 1 tbsp coriander leaves: chopped.
- 1/4 cup of paneer cheese

## Instructions:

Heat oil and add mustard seed to a saucepan. When seeds splutter, add salt, chili, and semolina. Roast until slightly brown, semolina rises. Remove from the heat and allow it cool. Mix the yogurt with water and whisk until creamy. Add paneer, Corn, yogurt, and cilantro to the cooled semolina mixture. Blend well and for 10 minutes, set aside. Grease with ghee (clarified butter) on the Idli mold and spoon small batter portions into the mold. Steam and cook for 10 minutes, then remove it from the mold. Sprinkle with cilantro that has been finely sliced and served with Cilantro Chutney.

## 98- Cucumbers with Sour Cream

Preparation time: 20-30 minutes

Cooking Time: 0 minutes

Servings: 4

Difficulty Level: Easy

### Nutritional Information:

Calories: 64 kcal, protein: 1 g, carbohydrates: 4 g, Fat: 5 g, Cholesterol: 3 mg, Fiber: 0.8 g, Sodium: 72 mg, Potassium: 113 mg, Phosphorus: 24 mg, Calcium: 21 mg

### Ingredients:

- 1/8 teaspoon of salt
- 2 medium cucumbers
- 1/4 cup of white wine vinegar
- 1/2 medium sweet onion
- 1 tablespoon of canola oil
- 1/2 cup of reduced-fat sour cream
- 1/8 teaspoon of black pepper

### Instructions:

Cucumbers are peeled, finely sliced, and placed in a medium-sized dish. Sprinkle salt on top. For 15 minutes, let it rest before rinsing and pressing away the extra moisture. Onions are thinly sliced. Toss in the remaining ingredients with the cucumbers. Before serving, chill in the refrigerator.

## 99- Jicama and Carrots

Preparation time: 10 minutes

Cooking Time: 0 minutes

Servings: 4

Difficulty Level: Easy

### Nutritional Information:

Calories: 75 kcal, protein: 1 g, carbohydrates: 11 g, Fat: 3 g, Cholesterol: 0 mg, Fiber: 2.8 g, Sodium: 12 mg, Potassium: 130 mg, Phosphorus: 15 mg, Calcium: 12 mg

### Ingredients:

- 3 tbsp lime juice
- 1 medium jicama
- 3 tbsp lemon juice
- 1 large carrot
- 1/3 cup of fresh basil leaves
- 1/2 red onion: medium
- 2 tbsp of apple cider vinegar
- 1-1/2 cup of seedless grapes

### Instructions:

Strip carrot and Jicama and split both into 1/4-inch sticks. Place them in a medium bowl. Dice the red onion and add it to the carrot/ jicama mixture. Halve the grapes and add them to the vegetables. Split the basil leaves and add them to the bowl. Drizzle other ingredients with lemon juice and. apple cider vinegar. Before serving, cool it and mix it properly.

## 100- Wonton Quiche Minis

Preparation time: 10 minutes

Cooking Time: 15-20 minutes

Servings: 12

Difficulty Level: Medium

### Nutritional Information:

Calories: 70 kcal, protein: 4 g, carbohydrates: 8 g, Fat: 2 g, Cholesterol: 91 mg, Fiber: 0.2 g, Sodium: 95 mg, Potassium: 47 mg, Phosphorus: 55 mg, Calcium: 16 mg

## Ingredients:

- 2 tablespoons of green onions
- 1-ounce cooked lean ham
- 5 large eggs
- 2 tablespoons of sweet red pepper
- 24 wonton wrappers; (3-1/4" x 3")
- 1 tablespoon of all-purpose white flour

## Instructions:

Set the oven to 350° F. Slice the ham finely. Chop red pepper &green onions. Eggs, onions, pepper, ham, and flour are mixed well in a medium bowl before placing aside. Sprinkle cooking spray on 24 little muffin tins/cups. Each cup is lined by gently pushing the center of one wonton wrapper into it, allowing the ends to hang over the cup's sides. Divide the egg mixture equally among the 24 wonton-lined cups before spooning it. For about 12 to 15 minutes, bake it until a toothpick inserted close to the middle comes out clean.

# CHAPTER 6

## Appetizer Recipes

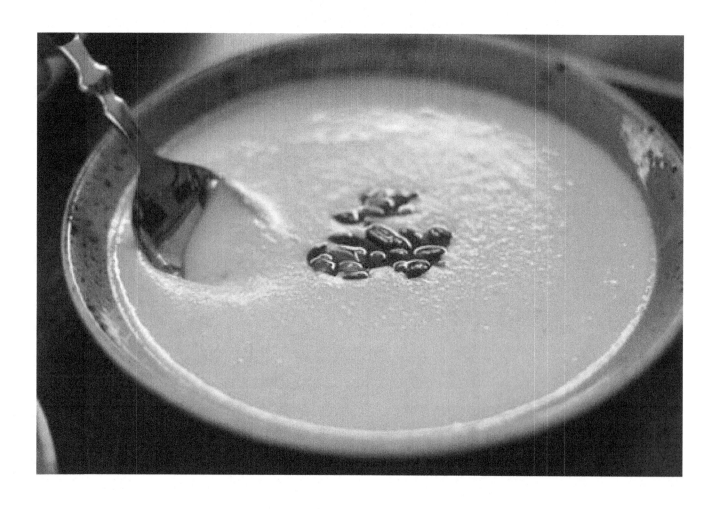

# 101- Cream of Water Cress

Preparation time: 10 minutes

Cooking Time: 50 minutes

Servings: 4

Difficulty Level: Medium

## Nutritional Information:

Calories: 189.9 kcal, protein: 4.4 g, carbohydrates: 14.3 g, Fat: 13.3 g, Cholesterol: 44.1 mg, Fiber: 1.4 g, Sodium: 89.4 mg, Potassium: 527 mg, Phosphorus: 355 mg, Calcium: 75 mg

## Ingredients:

- Black pepper: freshly ground.
- ½ tsp of olive oil
- 6 garlic cloves
- 1 tsp butter: unsalted
- 4 cups watercress: chopped.
- ½ sweet onion, chopped.
- ¼ cup of fresh parsley: chopped.
- ¼ cup of heavy cream
- 3 cups of water
- 1 tbsp lemon juice: freshly squeezed.

## Instructions:

Preheat the oven to 400°F. On a piece of aluminum foil, put the garlic. Drizzle the foil with the olive oil and roll it into a small packet. Put that packet in a pie dish and cook the garlic for around 20 minutes or until very tender. Take the garlic from the oven; cool it aside. In a wide saucepan over medium to high heat, melt the butter. Sauté the onion until tender, or around 4 minutes. Add the cress and parsley and sauté for five minutes. Mix in the water and the pulp of the roasted garlic. Boil the broth, then reduce the heat to a low amount.

Simmer the broth until the vegetables are soft or for around 20 minutes. Cool the soup for approximately 5 minutes, then blend it with the heavy cream to make a puree. Shift the soup to the pot and put it on low heat until it is warmed. Season with pepper and add lemon juice.

# 102- Mexican Nibbles

Preparation time: 5 minutes

Cooking Time: 20 minutes

Servings: 6

Difficulty Level: Easy

## Nutritional Information:

Calories: 312 kcal, protein: 6 g, carbohydrates: 52 g, Fat: 9 g, Cholesterol: 0 mg, Fiber: 3 g, Sodium: 97 mg, Potassium: 340 mg, Phosphorus: 107 mg, Calcium: 49 mg

## Ingredients:

- 2½ tsp. of chili powder
- 1 egg white: room temperature
- ½ tsp. of cumin
- 3 cups cereal
- ¼ tsp. of garlic powder

## Instructions:

Beat the egg white until it is foamy. In the dish, combine chili powder, cumin, and garlic powder, mix well, and pour it into the egg white. Simply add cereal and mix to cover softly. Layer the mixture over a thinly greased sheet. At 325°F, bake it for 15 minutes, keep stirring every 5 minutes, and serve it cool or store.

# 103- Baked Garlic

Preparation time: 5 minutes

Cooking Time: 25 minutes

Servings: 20

Difficulty Level: Easy

## Nutritional Information:

Calories: 33 kcal, protein: 0 g, carbohydrates: 2 g, Fat: 3 g, Cholesterol: 0 mg, Fiber: 0.1 g, Sodium: 1 mg, Potassium: 26 mg, Phosphorus: 9 mg, Calcium: 11 mg

## Ingredients:

- Toasted bread (French bread or baguette)
- Small, covered baking dish
- 4 whole bulbs or heads of garlic
- 1 tsp. of oregano or rosemary: dried
- 1 tbsp. of olive oil

## Instructions:

Preheat the oven to 375°F. To expose cloves, cut the tops off the garlic bulbs (around 1/2"). Bake wrapped for one hour, basting regularly. Spray with oil and season with herbs. Squeeze the garlic from the skin and eat it. Spread or use as a basis for wonderful sauces on your favorite crusty bread.

## 104- Creamy Cucumber

Preparation time: 10 minutes

Cooking Time: 0 minutes

Servings: 2

Difficulty Level: Easy

## Nutritional Information:

Calories: 94 kcal, protein: 1 g, carbohydrates: 9 g, Fat: 6g, Cholesterol: 16 mg, Fiber: 0.5 g, Sodium: 26 mg, Potassium: 125 mg, Phosphorus: 47 mg, Calcium: 43 mg

## Ingredients:

- 1 medium cucumber, finely minced, peeled, and seeded.
- 1/2-pound of cream cheese: softened.
- 1/2 tbsp. of minced onion

- 1/2 tbsp. of mayonnaise
- 1/4 tsp. of salt
- 1/8 tsp. of food coloring: green

## Instructions:

Add the cream cheese, onion, mayonnaise, salt, and food coloring into a mixing container. Blend smoothly. To the onion mixture, add the cucumber and stir them.

## 105- Dill Nibbles

Preparation time: 10 minutes

Cooking Time: 40 minutes

Servings: 30

Difficulty Level: Medium

## Nutritional Information:

Calories: 116 kcal, protein: 2 g, carbohydrates: 18 g, Fat: 4 g, Cholesterol: 9 mg, Fiber: 0.4 g, Sodium: 217 mg, Potassium: 45 mg, Phosphorus: 34 mg, Calcium: 96 mg

## Ingredients:

- 5 tbsp. of butter, unsalted
- 1- and 3/4 pounds of Chex cereal Rice
- 3/4-pound of Chex cereal Corn
- 1 and 1/2 tsp. of garlic powder
- 1 medium Parmesan cheese
- 3 tsp. of Dill weed, dried.
- 1/2 tbsp. of Worcestershire sauce

## Instructions:

Preheat the oven to 250 deg. F. In a large baking pan, add the rice and corn cereal. Place the pot over medium-low heat and place the unsalted butter at the base of the pot. Heat until it melts. Add the melted butter to the Worcestershire sauce, parmesan cheese, dill weed, and garlic powder. Stir well. Add a quarter of the melted butter mixture to the baking pan over the rice and corn cereal. Mix evenly to coat. Put them in the oven and bake for 15 minutes. Take the cereal mixture out of the oven and add the melted butter mixture to the cereal mixture. Thoroughly mix. Transfer the pan back to the oven. Bake for 15 more minutes. Repeat steps 7 to 9 twice or before all the melted butter mixture is mixed. Continue to cook for about 1 hour or until crispy.

# 106- Spicy Eggs

Preparation time: 10 minutes

Cooking Time: 0 minutes

Servings: 6

Difficulty Level: Medium

## Nutritional Information:

Calories: 240 kcal, protein: 15 g, carbohydrates: 9 g, Fat: 17 g, Cholesterol: 80 mg, Fiber: 3 g, Sodium: 194 mg, Potassium: 450 mg, Phosphorus: 650 mg, Calcium: 121 mg

## Ingredients:

- 1 tbsp. Of canned pimento, diced.
- 2 large, hard-boiled eggs (cooled and peeled).
- 1/2 tsp. of mustard, dry
- 2 tbsp. of mayonnaise
- 1/8 tsp. of paprika
- 1/2 tsp. of black pepper

## Instructions:

Cut eggs in half and remove the yolk. Add the pimento, yolk, mayonnaise, pepper, and vinegar to a mixing dish. Mix well to blend. Equally, put the yolk mixture in the white parts of the egg, and spread the paprika over the white parts.

# 107- Fresh Fruit Cranberry Dip

Preparation time: 10 minutes

Cooking Time: 0 minutes

Servings: 24

Difficulty Level: Easy

## Nutritional Information:

Calories: 70 kcal, protein: 0 g, carbohydrates: 13 g, Fat: 2 g, Cholesterol: 4 mg, Fiber: 1.5 g, Sodium: 8 mg, Potassium: 101 mg, Phosphorus: 15 mg, Calcium: 17 mg

## Ingredients:

- 8 pineapples: medium, fresh, cut into chunks.
- 1/4 tsp. of ginger, ground
- 5 tbsp. of cranberry sauce, whole berry
- 1/2 pound of sour cream
- 1/4 tsp. of nutmeg
- 4 pears: medium sliced into 12 chunks.
- 1/2 tbsp. of lemon juice
- 4 apples: medium, sliced into 12 chunks.

## Instructions:

Place the ginger, cranberry sauce, nutmeg, and sour cream in a food processor. Process well. To a bowl, shift the mixture. To avoid discoloration, add the lemon juice with the pears and apple slices. Place the lemon pineapple, apples, and pears on a tray and the processed cranberry sauce mixture bowl in the center. Freeze the fruit before serving with the dip.

# 108- Barbecue Meatballs

Preparation time: 10 minutes

Cooking Time: 20 minutes

Servings: 24

Difficulty Level: Medium

## Nutritional Information:

Calories: 176 kcal, protein: 11 g, carbohydrates: 6 g, Fat: 12 g, Cholesterol: 55 mg, Fiber: 0.5 g, Sodium: 180 mg, Potassium: 208 mg, Phosphorus: 107 mg, Calcium: 24 mg

## Ingredients:

- 3 pounds of ground beef
- 1/2 cup of onion
- 1/2 cup of rice milk, unenriched
- 2 large eggs
- 1 tbsp of dried thyme
- 1 cup of oatmeal, uncooked
- 1/2 tsp of pepper
- 1 tsp of dried oregano
- 1/3 cup of water
- 1 cup of barbecue sauce

## Instructions:

Preheat the oven to 375° F. Slice the onions and beat the eggs. Mix all ingredients in a large bowl, except for the barbecue sauce and water. Place on a baking sheet and roll into 1-inch balls. Bake for 15 minutes until the meatballs are fully cooked. Combine water and barbecue sauce at low temperatures in a warming dish or Crockpot. Add and stir the meatballs. Cover until having to serve.

## 109- Seasoning Dip

Preparation time: 5 minutes ( Freeze: 4 hours)

Cooking Time: 0 minutes

Servings: 8

Difficulty Level: Easy

## Nutritional Information:

Calories: 78 kcal, protein: 1 g, carbohydrates: 1 g, Fat: 8 g, Cholesterol: 13 mg, Fiber: 0.8 g, Sodium: 51 mg, Potassium: 30 mg, Phosphorus: 25 mg, Calcium: 25 mg

## Ingredients:

- 1/2 tbsp. of Worcestershire sauce, low-sodium
- 5 tbsp. of sour cream
- 1 and 1/2 tsp. of herb seasoning blend, salt-free
- 5 tbsp. of plain Greek yogurt, non-fat

## Instructions:

Add the worcestershire sauce, sour cream, herb seasoning, and greek yogurt to a small mixing bowl and mix it well. Cover and freeze it for 4 hours and then stir to serve.

## 110- Bean Dip

Preparation time: 10 minutes

Cooking Time: 10 minutes

Servings: 15-16

Difficulty Level: Medium

## Nutritional Information:

Calories: 64 kcal, protein: 2 g, carbohydrates: 5 g, Fat: 4 g, Cholesterol: 7 mg, Fiber: 0.9 g, Sodium: 72 mg, Potassium: 73 mg, Phosphorus: 33 mg, Calcium: 26 mg

## Ingredients:

- 1 bell pepper: green
- 1/2 red onion: large
- fresh cilantro: 1/3 cup
- white hominy: 2-1/2 cups
- 1 red bell pepper
- 8 ounces of cream cheese: low-fat
- 3 garlic cloves
- 1/4 cup of olive oil
- Cooked pinto beans: 1 cup.
- 1/4 tsp of chili powder
- 1 tbsp of ground cumin
- 1 lime
- Twelve ounces sour cream: low-fat.

## Instructions:

Cut the onion, cilantro, and bell peppers. In a food processor, combine pinto beans, hominy, low-fat cream cheese, 2 cloves of garlic, olive oil, chili powder, and cumin. Spread into a 9 " x 9" pan. Layer the sour cream over the bean mixture with a spatula. Red cabbage, green and red bell peppers, and 1 clove of garlic, finely sauté in a pan. For peppers to be firm, not mushy, stop overcooking. For extra flavor, squeeze the lime over the sautéed bell pepper and onion mixture and then remove the excess oil. Spoon the bell pepper mixture on top of the sour cream and smooth until coated with dip.

## 111- Summer Fruit Dip

Preparation time: 5 minutes

Cooking Time: 0 minutes

Servings: 15

Difficulty Level: Easy

### Nutritional Information:

Calories: 90 kcal, protein: 1 g, carbohydrates: 10 g, Fat: 5 g, Cholesterol: 17 mg, Fiber: 0 g, Sodium: 55 mg, Potassium: 19 mg, Phosphorus: 17 mg, Calcium: 13 mg

### Ingredients:

- 7 ounces of marshmallow cream
- 8 ounces cream cheese: low-fat

### INSTRUCTIONS:

Use an electric processor to combine the marshmallow completely and softened cream cheese. Enjoy kidney-friendly fruits such as mango, grapes, strawberries, and apples for dipping.

## 112- Brown Sugar Apple Dip

Preparation time: 25 minutes

Cooking Time: 0 minutes

Servings: 8

Difficulty Level: Easy

### Nutritional Information:

Calories: 154 kcal, protein: 2 g, carbohydrates: 14 g, Fat: 10 g, Cholesterol: 31 mg, Fiber: 0 g, Sodium: 107 mg, Potassium: 57 mg, Phosphorus: 31 mg, Calcium: 39 mg

### Ingredients:

- 1/2 tsp of vanilla extract
- 3/4 cup of brown sugar, unpacked.
- 8 ounces of cream cheese

### Instructions:

Put aside the cream cheese to melt for 20 minutes at room temperature. Mix the brown sugar, vanilla, and cream cheese, until fully combined, with a hand-held mixer. Enjoy sliced apple.

## 113- Hot Crab Dip

Preparation time: 10 minutes

Cooking Time: 15 minutes

Servings: 10

Difficulty Level: Medium

### Nutritional Information:

Calories: 96 kcal, protein: 8 g, carbohydrates: 1 g, Fat: 8 g, Cholesterol: 42 mg, Fiber: 0 g, Sodium: 191 mg, Potassium: 92 mg, Phosphorus: 68 mg, Calcium: 43 mg

### Ingredients:

- 1 tbsp of minced onion
- 8 ounces cream cheese
- 2 tsp of Worcestershire sauce
- 1 tsp of lemon juice

- 1/8 tsp of cayenne pepper
- 1/8 tsp of black pepper
- 6 ounces crab meat: canned
- 2 tbsp 1% low-fat milk

## Instructions:

Set the oven to 375º F. Place the cream cheese to melt. Mince the onion finely. Place melted cream cheese in a dish. Add the lemon juice, onion, Worcestershire sauce, cayenne pepper, and black pepper. Mix thoroughly. Stir the milk in. Then add crab meat and whisk until mixed. Place this mixture into an oven-safe dish. Then bake it uncovered for 15 minutes, until hot and fluffy.

## 114- Garden Veggie Dip

Preparation time: 20 minutes

Cooking Time: 0 minutes

Servings: 20

Difficulty Level: Medium

### Nutritional Information:

Calories: 82 kcal, protein: 2 g, carbohydrates: 5 g, Fat: 6 g, Cholesterol: 17 mg, Fiber: 1.2 g, Sodium: 88 mg, Potassium: 208 mg, Phosphorus: 42 mg, Calcium: 39 mg

### Ingredients:

- 1/4 cup of radish
- 8 ounces cream cheese
- 1/4 cup of green pepper
- 2 cucumbers: medium
- 1/4 cup of green onion
- 4 carrots: medium
- 1/4 cup of green onion
- 7 celery stalks
- 1/2 tsp of herb seasoning mix
- 1/4 cup of cucumber
- 3 red bell peppers: medium
- 1 cup of sour cream

- 1/4 tsp of salt
- 3 green bell peppers: medium
- 1 tbsp of sugar

## Instructions:

Set out the cream cheese to melt it. Chop the radish, green onion, green pepper, and 1/4 cup of the cucumber. Then drain the cucumber. Cut the celery and carrots into sticks and bell peppers into strips with the remaining 2 cucumber slices. On a serving tray, place the vegetables. Put the sour cream, cream cheese, green onion, radish, 1/4 cup chopped cucumber, sugar, 1/4 cup chopped green pepper, salt, and herbs in a big mixing bowl. Mix using an electric mixer at low speed for around 1 minute until well blended. Spoon it into a dish for serving.

## 115- Artichoke Dip

Preparation time: 10 minutes

Cooking Time: 40 minutes

Servings: 8

Difficulty Level: Medium

### Nutritional Information:

Calories: 40 kcal, protein: 1 g, carbohydrates: 4 g, Fat: 2.4 g, Cholesterol: 5 mg, Fiber: 1.5 g, Sodium: 113 mg, Potassium: 75 mg, Phosphorus: 31 mg, Calcium: 24 mg

### Ingredients:

- 1 tbsp Parmesan cheese
- 1/4 cup of mayonnaise
- 1 cup of artichoke hearts: frozen
- 2 tbsp of cream cheese
- 1/4 cup of sour cream
- 2 tsp of hot sauce
- 1 large garlic clove

## Instructions:

Preheat the oven to 375º F. In a saucepan, put the artichoke hearts, cover them with water, and bring them to a boil. Lower the heat to medium and simmer for around 6 minutes. Sewer and rinse with water to cool. Slice Artichoke hearts. Combine the whipped cream, mayonnaise, cloves of garlic, cream cheese, and crushed spicy sauce in a medium dish. Add the artichoke and stir to blend. Move the mixture to a tray for baking. Cover with Parmesan cheese. Put in the oven and cook for 30 minutes until the top is bubbly.

## 116- Holiday Cheese Ball

Preparation time: 40 minutes

Cooking Time: 0 minutes

Servings: 12

Difficulty Level: Easy

## Nutritional Information:

Calories: 140 kcal, protein: 2 g, carbohydrates: 4 g, Fat: 13 g, Cholesterol: 24 mg, Fiber: 0.3 g, Sodium: 131 mg, Potassium: 55 mg, Phosphorus: 32 mg, Calcium: 6 mg

## Ingredients:

- 1/4 cup of Russian salad dressing
- 8 ounces of cream cheese
- 1/3 cup of finely ground walnuts
- 1 tsp of onion powder

## Instructions:

Melt the cream cheese. Mix the salad dressing, onion powder, and cream cheese in a medium dish. Put it in the fridge to cool for 30 minutes. Shape the mixture of cheese into a ball. Place the ground walnuts on a plate and roll to cover the cheese puck. Cover and chill the cheese ball in plastic wrap before ready to eat.

## 117- Hula Meatballs

Preparation time: 10 minutes

Cooking Time: 20-30 minutes

Servings: 12

Difficulty Level: Medium

## Nutritional Information:

Calories: 200 kcal, protein: 11 g, carbohydrates: 16 g, Fat: 10 g, Cholesterol: 72 mg, Fiber: 0.5 g, Sodium: 92 mg, Potassium: 189 mg, Phosphorus: 84 mg, Calcium: 14 mg

## Ingredients:

- 4 tbsp of onion
- 4 large eggs
- 7 tbsp of cornstarch
- 1/2 tsp of nutmeg
- 2 cups of bell peppers (red and green)
- 3 pounds of ground beef
- 2 tbsp low-sodium soy sauce.
- 1/2 tsp of garlic powder
- 1/2 cup of white sugar
- 2/3 cup of water
- 1/3 cup of vinegar
- 1/2 cup of brown sugar
- Canned pineapple chunks: 40 ounces
- 2 cups of pineapple juice

## Instructions:

Preheat the oven to 375 degrees F. Smash bell peppers and onion. Combine 1 tablespoon of cornstarch, carrot, black pepper, nutmeg, garlic powder, ground beef, and eggs. Mix thoroughly. Shape into 1-inch balls and put on a baking sheet. Bake for 10 minutes until the meatballs are thoroughly cooked. Drain the pineapple juice into a measuring cup. To make 2 cups, add water.

Combine the remaining 6 teaspoons of cornstarch, vinegar, reduced-sodium soy sauce, unpacked brown sugar, water, white sugar, and Pineapple juice. Heat until it thickens; continuously stir it. Remove from the heat. In a covered heating dish or Crockpot placed on a low setting, put meatballs, gravy, pineapple bits, and green and red peppers until ready to serve.

# 118- Honey-Maple Trail Mix

Preparation time: 10 minutes

Cooking Time: 45 minutes

Servings: 12

Difficulty Level: Medium

## Nutritional Information:

Calories: 262 kcal, protein: 3 g, carbohydrates: 47 g, Fat: 9 g, Cholesterol: 11 mg, Fiber: 1.8 g, Sodium: 178 mg, Potassium: 84 mg, Phosphorus: 66 mg, Calcium: 63 mg

## Ingredients:

- 5 ounces of cranberries (dried, sweetened).
- 3 cups of Golden Graham cereal
- Cinnamon snack cookies: 10 ounces
- 5 cups of Rice Chex cereal
- 1/2 cup of unsalted butter
- Pretzel Crisps: 6 ounces
- 1/4 cup of honey
- Crispy Apple Chips; 3 ounces
- 1/3 cup of dark brown sugar
- 1/4 cup of maple syrup

## Instructions:

Combine Rice Chex, Golden Graham's cereals, and pretzels in a big bowl. In a shallow saucepan, melt the butter and add the brown sugar, maple syrup, and honey. Cook until the sugar is melted over low heat. Pour over the cereal mixture and blend properly before all the pieces have been covered. Preheat the oven to 325 degrees F. Spray the foil with cooking spray and make 3

jelly roll pans lined with aluminum foil. Spread over pans the cereal mixture evenly. Bake for 20 minutes at 325 ° F; stirring halfway once. Mix the cranberries and apple chips; split and stir equally between the dishes. Bake for another 5 minutes; cool fully and put in an airtight jar.

# 119- Holiday Tuna Ball

Preparation time: 50 minutes

Cooking Time: 0 minutes

Servings: 16

Difficulty Level: Easy

## Nutritional Information:

Calories: 77 kcal, protein: 3 g, carbohydrates: 5 g, Fat: 5 g, Cholesterol: 18 mg, Fiber: 0.3 g, Sodium: 92 mg, Potassium: 51 mg, Phosphorus: 38 mg, Calcium: 20 mg

## Ingredients:

- canned tuna: 5 ounces
- cream cheese: 8 ounces
- 1/4 cup of celery
- 1/3 cup of dried cranberries: sweetened
- 1/4 tsp of ground cumin
- 2 tbsp red onion
- 1 tbsp dried parsley
- 1/4 cup dry breadcrumbs

## Instructions

Place the cream cheese out for 30 minutes to melt. Use a fork to drain canned tuna and flake it. Combine the cream cheese, salmon, cranberries, celery, cumin, and onion in a mixing bowl. When well mixed, blend with an electric mixer. The parsley and breadcrumbs are mixed and then placed on a tray. Form cream cheese mix into a puck and roll it to coat it with breadcrumbs. Cover and refrigerate the ball in plastic wrap before ready to eat.

## 120- Italian Meatballs

Preparation time: 10 minutes

Cooking Time: 20 minutes

Servings: 12

Difficulty Level: Medium

### Nutritional Information:

Calories: 160 kcal, protein: 12 g, carbohydrates: 3 g, Fat: 11 g, Cholesterol: 65 mg, Fiber: 0.5 g, Sodium: 54 mg, Potassium: 133 mg, Phosphorus: 99 mg, Calcium: 27 mg

### Ingredients:

- 3 large eggs
- 1 cup of onion
- 1 tbsp garlic powder
- ground beef: 3 pounds
- 1 tbsp of olive oil
- 1 cup of oatmeal, uncooked
- 6 tbsp of parmesan cheese
- 1 tsp black pepper: ground
- 2 tsp oregano, dried
- 1 cup of Roasted Red Pepper Tomato Sauce

### Instructions:

Make a Roasted Red Pepper Tomato Sauce and put it aside. Preheat the oven to 375° F and cut onions. In a large bowl, beat the eggs, add all the ingredients, and blend. Put on a baking sheet and roll into 1-inch balls. Bake for 15 minutes, till the meatballs, are thoroughly cooked. To serve, put meatballs on a low heat setting in a cooking pan or slow cooker. Serve with sauce and noodles.

## 121- Crab-Stuffed Celery Logs

Preparation time: 15 minutes

Cooking Time: 0 minutes

Servings: 4

Difficulty Level: Medium

### Nutritional Information:

Calories: 34 kcal, protein: 2 g, carbohydrates: 2 g, Fat: 2 g, Cholesterol: 9 mg, Fiber: 0.7 g, Sodium: 94 mg, Potassium: 134 mg, Phosphorus: 31 mg, Calcium: 25 mg

### Ingredients:

- 1 tbsp red onion
- 1/4 cup of crab meat
- 4 celery ribs (medium 8-inch)
- 1/4 tsp paprika
- 2 tsp mayonnaise
- 1/2 tsp lemon juice

### Instructions:

Chop the ends of the celery rib. Drain the crab meat and flake it. Just mince the onion. Combine the crab meat, cabbage, lemon juice, and mayonnaise in a shallow dish. Using 1 tablespoon of the crab mix, fill each celery rib. Break each rib of celery into 3 parts. Before eating, dust the crab-stuffed celery bits with paprika.

## 122- Raspberry Wings

Preparation time: 5 minutes

Cooking Time: 40 minutes

Servings: 12

Difficulty Level: Medium

### Nutritional Information:

Calories: 200 kcal, protein: 11 g, carbohydrates: 21 g, Fat: 8 g, Cholesterol: 34 mg, Fiber: 0.7 g, Sodium: 181 mg, Potassium: 121 mg, Phosphorus: 70 mg, Calcium: 7 mg

## Ingredients:

- 3 tbsp low-sodium soy sauce.
- 24 chicken wing drumettes
- 2 cups of raspberry jam
- 1/3 cup of balsamic vinegar

## Instruction:

Preheat the oven to 400° F. Heat the jam, vinegar, and soy sauce in a saucepan, and stir until smooth. In a wide bowl, place the wings. Spread the jam sauce over the wings and heavily cover them with a flip. Spray cooking spray on a broad baking dish and put the chicken wings. For 30 to 35 minutes, roast them. Serve the wings warm or put on a low setting in a covered warming dish or Crockpot until ready to serve.

## 123- Chili Lime Dip

Preparation time: 40 minutes

Cooking Time: 0 minutes

Servings: 8

Difficulty Level: Easy

### Nutritional Information:

Calories: 38 kcal, protein: 1 g, carbohydrates: 1.5 g, Fat: 3 g, Cholesterol: 4 mg, Fiber: 0.2 g, Sodium: 25 mg, Potassium: 51 mg, Phosphorus: 15 mg, Calcium: 5.5 mg

### Ingredients:

- 2 tbsp of mayonnaise
- 1/2 cup of silken tofu
- 1 tsp of chili powder
- 3 tbsp fresh cilantro: chopped.
- 1/2 cup of roasted red peppers
- 1 tsp of onion powder
- 1 1/2 tbsp of lime juice

## Instructions:

Place all the ingredients in a food processor and blend for around 30 seconds until smooth. In a shallow bowl, pour it, cover, and refrigerate for at least 30 minutes.

## 124- Tortilla Rollups

Preparation time: 15 minutes

Cooking Time: 0 minutes

Servings: 4

Difficulty Level: Medium

### Nutritional Information:

Calories: 223 kcal, protein: 10 g, carbohydrates: 21 g, Fat: 11 g, Cholesterol: 39 mg, Fiber: 1.7 g, Sodium: 298 mg, Potassium: 199 mg, Phosphorus: 126 mg, Calcium: 58 mg

### Ingredients:

- 2 tbsp of pimento
- 1/2 cup of raw spinach leaves
- 2 tbsp onion
- 3 ounces cooked turkey breast; unprocessed
- 1/2 cup of crushed Pineapple
- 2 burrito size flour tortillas,
- 1 tsp of herb seasoning blend
- 1/2 cup of cream cheese: whipped.

### Instructions:

Dice the turkey breast pimento and onion, chop spinach and drain Pineapple. Scatter cream cheese on each tortilla for coating, then sprinkle with herb seasoning. Put the remainder of the ingredients in a container and blend. Divide the mixture into 2 parts. Place half of the tortillas on each one and roll up like a jelly roll. Cut the ends and split each roll into 6 parts.

## 125- Asian Eggplant Dip

Preparation time: 5 minutes

Cooking Time: 50 minutes

Servings: 4-5

Difficulty Level: Medium

### Nutritional Information:

Calories: 60 kcal, protein: 1.3 g, carbohydrates: 11 g, Fat: 1.8 g, Cholesterol: 0 mg, Fiber: 3 g, Sodium: 11 mg, Potassium: 262 mg, Phosphorus: 31 mg, Calcium: 30 mg

### Ingredients:

- 2 tbsp of brown sugar
- 1 large eggplant
- 1 tbsp of rice vinegar
- 4 cloves garlic finely chopped.
- 1 tbsp of water
- 1 tsp of sesame oil
- 1 tsp of vegetable oil
- 4 green onions, chopped.
- 1 tbsp of fresh ginger root: finely chopped.
- 2 tbsp of fresh cilantro: chopped.
- 1 tsp of chili paste.

### Instructions:

Bake the eggplant in a preheated oven at 425 ° F for around 45 minutes. Peel the eggplants and finely chop them. Mix the vinegar, sugar, and water in a medium bowl. Sauté the ginger, garlic, green, chili paste, and onions in a wide pan until fragrant. Add a mixture of vinegar. Add the eggplant when it starts bubbling. Stir to blend. Remove from the heat and add the freshly minced cilantro and sesame oil. Serve at room temperature or cool.

## 126- Low Sodium Homemade Pesto

Preparation time: 10 minutes

Cooking Time: 0 minutes

Servings: 6

Difficulty Level: Easy

### Nutritional Information:

Calories: 141 kcal, protein: 1 g, carbohydrates: 1 g, Fat: 15 g, Cholesterol: 0 mg, Fiber: 1 g, Sodium: 98 mg, Potassium: 45 mg, Phosphorus: 87 mg, Calcium: 17 mg

### Ingredients:

- 1/4 cup of walnuts
- 1 1/2 cup of fresh basil leaves
- 1 clove garlic
- 1/3 cup of olive oil: extra virgin
- 1/4 tsp salt, to taste.
- 1–2 tsp lemon juice, to taste.
- Optional: 1-2 tbsp nutritional yeast, to taste
- 1/4 tsp pepper, to taste.

### Instructions:

Add all ingredients to the mixer, and blend at high speed until smoothness is achieved. Add seasonings to taste; for a cheesier flavor, add nutritional yeast. Pour the pesto into an airtight jar and store it for up to 5 days in the refrigerator or 30 days in the freezer.

## 127- Sour Cream Dip

Preparation time: 10 minutes

Cooking Time: 0 minutes

Servings: 8

Difficulty Level: Easy

### Nutritional Information:

Calories: 57 kcal, protein: <1 g, carbohydrates: 3 g, Fat: 6 g, Cholesterol: 17 mg, Fiber: 0 g,

Sodium: 9 mg, Potassium: 58 mg, Phosphorus: 23 mg, Calcium: 31 mg

## Ingredients:

- ½ tsp of onion powder
- sour cream: 8 ounces
- 1 tsp Worcestershire sauce: low sodium
- ½ tsp paprika
- 1 tbsp plus 1tsp Italian Seasoning Blend
- ½ tsp dried dill

## Instructions:

With a spoon, mix sour cream and all the spices, and let it stay overnight.

## 128- Vegan Kimchi

Preparation time: 20 minutes

Cooking Time: 0 minutes

Servings: 64

Difficulty Level: Medium

### Nutritional Information:

Calories: 160 kcal, protein: 6 g, carbohydrates: 11 g, Fat: 0.5 g, Cholesterol: 0 mg, Fiber: 4 g, Sodium: 111 mg, Potassium: 9 mg, Phosphorus: 2 mg, Calcium: 19 mg

### Ingredients:

- 4 stalks of green onions, only the green part, pieces
- 1 head napa cabbage; (1 lb.)
- 3 tbsp of red pepper flakes
- 4 cloves garlic; minced
- ½ cup of onions; thinly sliced
- 1-inch ginger; grated
- 2 tbsp of sea salt
- 1 tsp of sugar

## Instructions:

Cabbage is cut in 8 wedges vertically. Slices are placed in a big bowl. After 3–4 minutes, add 2 tablespoons of salt and massage it into the cabbage until it is moist and wilts. For 50 minutes, set it aside. Prepare the remaining ingredients in the meantime. Slice 1/2 cup of onions thinly. Green parts of onions are chopped into 2-inch chunks. Garlic cloves are minced. Fresh ginger is grated. Ginger and garlic are combined into a paste by adding 1 tsp sugar. After 50 minutes, put the cabbage into a colander and give it a good one-minute rinse under cold running water. For 30 minutes, drain the cabbage.

Add the chopped cabbage, green onion pieces, garlic ginger paste, sliced onions, and 3 tbsp. Of red pepper flakes to a large bowl. Mix well until combined. Fill clean jars with the mixture, leaving 1 inch of space at the top for fermentation. Place in the refrigerator for up to months for storage after three days on the counter at room temperature. In the refrigerator, the fermentation will continue to occur. After three days, the kimchi's top may seem frothy or include tiny bubbles, which indicates fermentation. Kimchi should be thrown out if it smells bad or appears slimy.

## 129- Roasted red pepper dip

Preparation time: 10 minutes

Cooking Time: 0 minutes

Servings: 4

Difficulty Level: Easy

### Nutritional Information:

Calories: 84 kcal, protein: 0.5 g, carbohydrates: 3 g, Fat: 8 g, Cholesterol: 0 mg, Fiber: 0.8 g, Sodium: 9 mg, Potassium: 89 mg, Phosphorus: 13 mg, Calcium: 20 mg

## Ingredients:

- 1 tsp of lemon juice
- 1 cup of roasted red peppers
- 1 tbsp of olive oil
- 1 tsp of cumin
- 1 clove garlic

## Instructions:

All ingredients are blended in a food processor. Serve with baked pita chips.

# 130- Baba Ghanouj

Preparation time: 10 minutes

Cooking Time: 30 minutes

Servings: 8

Difficulty Level: Medium

## Nutritional Information:

Calories: 51 kcal, protein: 1.0 g, carbohydrates: 5.0 g, Fat: 3.6 g, Cholesterol: 0 mg, Fiber: 2.4 g, Sodium: 2 mg, Potassium: 170 mg, Phosphorus: 22 mg, Calcium: 20 mg

## Ingredients:

- Lemon juice; to taste
- 1 large eggplant; lengthwise halved
- 2 tablespoons of olive oil
- 1 head of garlic; unpeeled

## Instructions:

Set an oven to 350°F with the center rack in place. Use parchment paper to cover a baking sheet. Lay the eggplant on the baking pan and cut the side down. Depending on the size of the eggplant, roast for about 1 hour or until the flesh is quite soft and readily separates from the skin. Let it cool. Trim the garlic cloves' tips in the meanwhile. In a piece of aluminum foil, put the cloves. To make a securely wrapped package, fold up and crimp the foil's edges. For approximately 20 minutes, roast the eggplant next to it until it is soft. Place it aside it let it cool. By running the cloves through a garlic press, purée them.

Scoop the eggplant's flesh with a spoon and put it in the food processor's bowl. Add the oil, lemon juice, and garlic purée until smooth. Use pepper to season. Serve with little pitas.

# CHAPTER 7

## Lunch Recipes

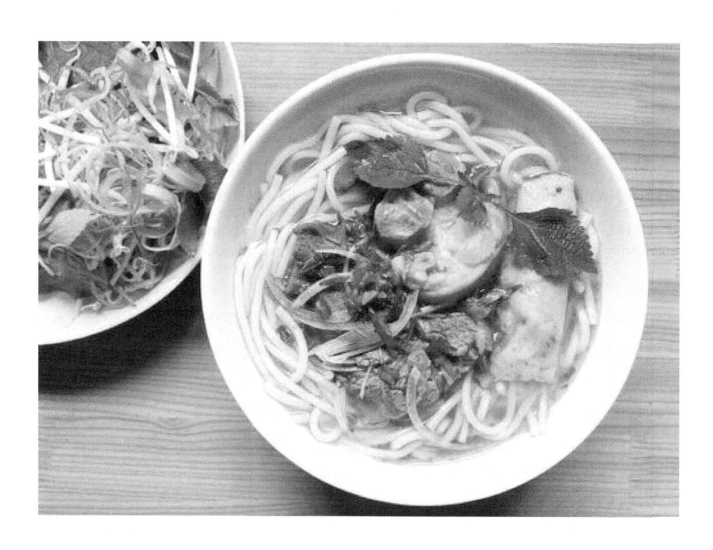

## 131- Veggie Strata

Preparation time: 1 hour 30 minutes

Cooking Time: 1 hour 40 minutes

Servings: 9

Difficulty Level: Easy

## Nutritional Information:

Calories: 212 kcal, protein: 11 g, carbohydrates: 15 g, Fat: 12 g, Cholesterol: 165 mg, Fiber: 2.0 g, Sodium: 218 mg, Potassium: 347 mg, Phosphorus: 207 mg, Calcium: 151 mg

## Ingredients:

- 7 slices of sourdough bread, 1/2" thick
- 1 tablespoon of unsalted margarine
- 7 large eggs
- 1 cup of raw mushrooms
- 1-3/4 cups of half & half creamer
- 15 spinach leaves: fresh
- 1 cup of red bell peppers
- 1 teaspoon of Worcestershire sauce
- 1 cup of onion
- 1/4 cup of tarragon vinegar
- 1 teaspoon of hot sauce
- 1-ounce shredded cheddar cheese
- 1/2 teaspoon of black pepper

## Instructions:

Cut bread into chunks and assemble on a baking sheet and bake for 15 minutes at 225° F. Flip the cubes and bake for another 15 minutes or until they are dry and crisp. Slice the bell peppers, mushrooms, and onion. Melt the margarine and sauté mushrooms, red peppers, and onion in a small skillet; with non-stick cooking spray, grease a 9-inch square baking dish. Layer bread cubes in the dish, sprinkle a mixture of vegetables, and place spinach on top. Then make a second layer in the same pattern. Add a mixture of black pepper, eggs, half & half creamer, hot sauce, Worcestershire sauce, and vinegar over the bread.

Use plastic wrap to cover the surface and refrigerate for at least 1 hour or overnight. Let it set for 20 minutes at room temperature. Uncover it and cook for 50 minutes. Scatter cheddar cheese over the top. Cook for an additional 10 minutes. Serve hot and cut into 9 servings.

## 132- Burritos with Pineapple Jalapeno Salsa

Preparation time: 10 minutes

Cooking Time: 10 minutes

Servings: 6

Difficulty Level: Medium

## Nutritional Information:

Calories: 414 kcal, protein: 19 g, carbohydrates: 44 g, Fat: 18 g, Cholesterol: 372 mg, Fiber: 3.8 g, Sodium: 546 mg, Potassium: 411 mg, Phosphorus: 325 mg, Calcium: 127 mg

## Ingredients:

- 12 large beaten eggs.
- 1 cup of green bell pepper, diced.
- 2 cups of fresh pineapple:1/2"-inch cubes.
- 2 jalapeno peppers: seeded and minced.
- 6 flour tortillas, 10" size
- 1 tablespoon of light brown sugar
- 3 tablespoons of fresh chopped cilantro.
- Two tablespoons of fresh lime juice
- 1 teaspoon of oil
- pepper to taste
- 1/4 cup of green onion, chopped.
- 1 cup of shitake or button sliced and chopped mushrooms.

## Instructions:

First, mix the cilantro, pineapple, lime juice, brown sugar, and jalapenos in a glass or ceramic dish to prepare the salsa, then set aside. Heat oil in a non-stick skillet and sauté the green peppers and mushrooms for 2 to 4 minutes over medium heat. Drain the excess liquid.

Pour the beaten eggs into a skillet over the mixture, and sprinkle the green onion evenly over the eggs. As the eggs begin to set, drag them with a spatula across the skillet, forming large curds. Until no apparent liquid or uncooked egg remains, cook and fold the eggs. Sprinkle pepper.

Spoon the mixture of eggs into individual tortillas. And cover each tortilla with 1/3 cup of pineapple salsa, fold the ends and fold burrito-style.

## 133- Huevos Rancheros

Preparation time: 5 minutes

Cooking Time: 15-20 minutes

Servings: 2

Difficulty Level: Easy

### Nutritional Information:

Calories: 320 kcal, protein: 9 g, carbohydrates: 19 g, Fat: 23 g, Cholesterol: 186 mg, Fiber: 3.7 g, Sodium: 146 mg, Potassium: 342 mg, Phosphorus: 200 mg, Calcium: 64 mg

### Ingredients:

- 2 corn tortillas
- 1/4 cup of onion
- 2 tablespoons of canola oil
- 1/2 cup of red chili sauce
- 2 large eggs
- 1/4 cup of bell peppers

## Instructions :

Cut bell pepper and onion. In a pan, heat 2 tablespoons of oil and crisp the tortillas on each side for around a minute or until they appear brown. Lay aside to drain on paper towels.

Sauté the bell pepper and onion in the same pan until tender. (If required, add additional oil.) Then remove them from the pan when cooked. Cook eggs, put one crisp tortilla on each tray, and cover it with eggs and sautéed vegetables. Serve with sauce and red chili.

Cook each side for around 2 minutes over medium heat. Turning the pancake when the top is bubbly and the sides are partially crisp. Avoid pressing with the spatula to keep the pancakes light and fluffy.

## 134  Chinese Hotdish

Preparation time: 25 minutes

Cooking Time: 1 hour 20 minutes

Servings: 8

Difficulty Level: Easy

### Nutritional Information:

Calories: 280 kcal, protein: 17 g, carbohydrates: 26 g, Fat: 12 g, Cholesterol: 44 mg, Fiber: 1.3 g, Sodium: 374 mg, Potassium: 339 mg, Phosphorus: 180 mg, Calcium: 34 mg

### Ingredients:

- 1-pound of lean ground beef
- 2 ribs celery
- 1 can (10.5-ounces) of Chicken Noodle Soup
- 1/2 cup of yellow onion
- 1 can (10.5-ounces) of Chicken Soup: Condensed Cream
- 2 cups of chow Mein noodles
- 1 tablespoon of low-sodium Worcestershire sauce.

- 2 cups of boiling water.
- 3/4 cup of rice, dry

## Instructions:

Preheat the oven to 350° F. Cut onion and celery. Cook ground beef, onion, and celery in a wide pan until brown. Transfer cooked beef to a casserole baking dish of 2 quarts in size. Use a wooden spoon to combine rice, chicken noodle broth, Worcestershire sauce, chicken soup cream, and hot water and blend completely, cover it. For 50 minutes, bake it. Take the bowl out of the oven and stir. Sprinkle the noodles over the casserole. Bake it again for 10 more minutes. Let it set before serving for 15 minutes.

## 135- Pasta Primavera

Preparation time: 5 minutes

Cooking Time: 10-15 minutes

Servings: 6

Difficulty Level: Easy

## Nutritional Information:

Calories: 273 kcal, protein: 13 g, carbohydrates: 48 g, Fat: 3 g, Cholesterol: 6 mg, Fiber: 4.5 g, Sodium: 115 mg, Potassium: 251 mg, Phosphorus: 154 mg, Calcium: 93 mg

## Ingredients:

- 2 tablespoons of white flour: all-purpose
- 1/4 cup of Parmesan cheese: grated.
- 12 ounces of pasta, uncooked
- 1/4 teaspoon of garlic powder
- 12 ounces of mixed vegetables: frozen
- 1/4 cup of half & half creamer
- 14 ounces of chicken broth: low-sodium

## Instructions:

In separate pans, cook vegetables and pasta according to package instructions. Skip salt. To a medium-sized stockpot, pour low sodium

chicken broth and cook over low heat. To prevent clumps formation, add flour to the whisking broth. Add garlic powder and half & half creamer; stir. Simmer for 5 to 10 minutes on low heat before the mixture thickens; stir occasionally. Add pasta and vegetables. Cook until thoroughly heated. Sprinkle and serve with Parmesan cheese.

## 136- Eggplant Casserole

Preparation time: 10 minutes

Cooking Time: 20 minutes

Servings: 4

Difficulty Level: Easy

## Nutritional Information:

Calories: 186 kcal, protein: 7 g, carbohydrates: 19 g, Fat: 9 g, Cholesterol: 124 mg, Fiber: 1.9 g, Sodium: 246 mg, Potassium: 224 mg, Phosphorus: 115 mg, Calcium: 56 mg

## Ingredients:

- 1 tablespoon of margarine
- 3 cups of eggplant
- 1/2 cup of liquid non-dairy creamer
- 3 large eggs
- 1/2 teaspoon of pepper
- 1/8 teaspoon of salt
- 1/2 cup of breadcrumbs
- 1/4 teaspoon of sage

## Instructions:

Preheat the oven to 350° F. Scrape and slice the eggplant. Add the pieces of eggplant to a saucepan, cover them with water and cook until tender. Mash it. Mix non-dairy creamer, beaten eggs, sage, salt, and pepper with mashed eggplant and pour this mixture into greased dish. Fold breadcrumbs with melted margarine. Add breadcrumbs over the casserole and bake for 20 minutes.

## 137- Savory White Rice

Preparation time: 10 minutes

Cooking Time: 30 minutes

Servings: 8

Difficulty Level: Easy

### Nutritional Information:

Calories: 84 kcal, protein: 4 g, carbohydrates: 17 g, Fat: 0 g, Cholesterol: 0 mg, Fiber: 0.5 g, Sodium: 40 mg, Potassium: 85 mg, Phosphorus: 42 mg, Calcium: 13 mg

### Ingredients:

- 2 cups of low-sodium chicken broth
- 1/3 cup of celery
- 1/2 teaspoon of black pepper
- 1/3 cup of green onion
- 1 teaspoon of margarine
- 1 cup of white rice, uncooked
- 1/3 cup of mushrooms

### Instructions:

Slice the green onion, mushrooms, and celery thinly. Add chicken broth and rice into a saucepan and bring it to boil over medium-high heat. Then add mushrooms, celery, and green onion. Press vegetables gently into the broth. Lower the heat and cover-up. Cook for 20 minutes or until the rice is soft and the broth is dried. Add pepper and margarine. Mix until it is covered with rice.

## 138- Zesty Chicken

Preparation time: 40 minutes

Cooking Time: 20-30 minutes

Servings: 2

Difficulty Level: Easy

### Nutritional Information:

Calories: 280 kcal, protein: 27 g, carbohydrates: 4 g, Fat: 16 g, Cholesterol: 73 mg, Fiber: 0.3 g, Sodium: 68 mg, Potassium: 280 mg, Phosphorus: 205 mg, Calcium: 26 mg

### Ingredients:

- 1/4 teaspoon of paprika
- 8 ounces of boneless, skinless chicken breast
- 1/4 cup of green onion
- 2 tablespoons of balsamic vinegar
- 1/2 teaspoon of garlic powder
- 2 tablespoons of olive oil
- 1/4 teaspoon of black pepper
- 1 teaspoon of fresh oregano

### Instructions:

Whisk together olive oil and balsamic vinegar in a measuring cup. Cut green onion and add it to seasonings and herbs. Mix it. Slice chicken into two chunks and add marinade to the chicken. Marinate and refrigerate for 30 minutes to 24 hours. Drain marinade from the chicken and fry both sides for several minutes in a medium-hot, non-stick, or greased skillet until fully fried.

## 139- Chicken and Watercress with Gratin Pasta

Preparation time: 10 minutes

Cooking Time: 50 minutes

Servings: 4

Difficulty Level: Medium

### Nutritional Information:

Calories: 345 kcal, protein: 19 g, carbohydrates: 38 g, Fat: 13 g, Cholesterol: 55 mg, Fiber: 2.1 g, Sodium: 437 mg, Potassium: 337 mg, Phosphorus: 248 mg, Calcium: 230 mg

## Ingredients:

- 1/2 cup of Parmesan cheese
- 2 cups of pasta spirals or shells
- 1/4 teaspoon of pepper
- 2 garlic cloves
- 1 tablespoon of olive oil
- 1 cup of fresh watercress
- 1 cup of cooked chicken: shredded.
- 1-2/3 cup of béchamel sauce (white sauce)

## Instructions:

According to the packet directions, cook pasta, and avoid using salt. Chop cloves of garlic, watercress, and onion. In a pan, heat oil and cook garlic and onion. Add watercress and chicken that is shredded. Mix and simmer until they are wilted with the watercress. Drain and add half of the béchamel sauce and chicken mixture. Cook pasta and mix thoroughly. To a baking dish coated with cooking spray, pour the mixture. Cover with béchamel sauce. Garnish Parmesan cheese and bake until golden brown for 30 to 40 minutes.

## 140- Macaroni and Cheese

Preparation time: 5 minutes

Cooking Time: 20-30 minutes

Servings: 4

Difficulty Level: Easy

## Nutritional Information:

Calories: 266 kcal, protein: 9 g, carbohydrates: 26 g, Fat: 14 g, Cholesterol: 43 mg, Fiber: 2.3 g, Sodium: 237 mg, Potassium: 222 mg, Phosphorus: 188 mg, Calcium: 147 mg

## Ingredients:

- 4 ounces of green chilies diced: canned or use fresh.

- 1/4 teaspoon of black pepper
- 1 cup of elbow pasta, uncooked
- 1 jar, 5 ounces of Pimento Cheese spread with cream cheese.

## Instructions:

Green chilies are rinsed. Cook elbow pasta without using salt or butter in boiling water until tender. Drain pasta. Add chilies and pimento cheese spread in them. Stir cooked and hot pasta until cheese melts. Add pepper to taste and serve it hot.

## 141- Spaghetti with Meat Sauce

Preparation time: 5 minutes

Cooking Time: 10 minutes

Servings: 8

Difficulty Level: Easy

## Nutritional Information:

Calories: 317 kcal, protein: 23 g, carbohydrates: 36 g, Fat: 9 g, Cholesterol: 58 mg, Fiber: 4.7 g, Sodium: 269 mg, Potassium: 538 mg, Phosphorus: 256 mg, Calcium: 52 mg

## Ingredients:

- 14 ounces of spaghetti sauce
- 1-1/2 pounds of ground beef
- 1 teaspoon of garlic powder
- 8 ounces of uncooked whole-wheat spaghetti,
- 1/3 cup of brown sugar
- 1 cup of onion
- 1 tablespoon of Italian Seasoning

## Instructions:

According to the box guidance, cook spaghetti, but skip the salt. Brown ground beef with onion in a large skillet and drain fat. Add garlic powder, brown sugar, and Italian seasonings. Stir in the spaghetti sauce and cook for 5 to 10 minutes.

Drain the spaghetti, then add it to the sauce. Mix it. Serve hot.

## 142- Garlic Mashed Potatoes

Preparation time: 10 minutes

Cooking Time: 20 minutes

Servings: 4

Difficulty Level: Easy

### Nutritional Information:

Calories: 185 kcal, protein: 2 g, carbohydrates: 15 g, Fat: 13 g, Cholesterol: 0 mg, Fiber: 0.7 g, Sodium: 103 mg, Potassium: 205 mg, Phosphorus: 65 mg, Calcium: 35 mg

### Ingredients:

- 1/4 cup of 1% low-fat milk
- 2 medium potatoes
- 1/4 cup of butter
- 2 garlic cloves

### Instructions:

Scrape and cut potatoes into small cubes. Boil garlic and potatoes until tender over medium heat. To reduce potassium, boil it twice. Then drain the water. Use a beater to mash garlic and potatoes, then add milk and butter until smoothly whipped.

## 143- Grilled Marinated Chicken

Preparation time: 2 hours 10 minutes

Cooking Time: 20-30 minutes

Servings: 4

Difficulty Level: Easy

### Nutritional Information:

Calories: 265 kcal, protein: 27 g, carbohydrates: 1 g, Fat: 17 g, Cholesterol: 73 mg, Fiber: 0.3 g,

Sodium: 65 mg, Potassium: 252 mg, Phosphorus: 200 mg, Calcium: 31 mg

### Ingredients:

- 1 garlic clove
- 4 skinless, boneless chicken breasts
- 1/4 cup of olive oil
- 1 teaspoon of onion powder
- 1/4 cup of red wine vinegar
- 1-1/2 teaspoon of Italian seasoning blend: dried
- fresh thyme sprigs (optional)
- 1/2 teaspoon of dried thyme

### Instructions:

Cut the chicken breasts in half, so each breast forms two thin fillets. Mince the garlic and mix properly with the remaining ingredients in a zip-top bag. To the bag, add the chicken fillets. Close and marinate for 2 hours or longer in the refrigerator, rotating periodically. Grill chicken over medium heat until it's done. If required, cover the chicken with fresh thyme sprigs while grilling, and turn the chicken just once.

## 144 Garlic Chicken with Balsamic Vinegar

Preparation time: 10 minutes

Cooking Time: 25 minutes

Servings: 4

Difficulty Level: Easy

### Nutritional Information:

Calories: 211 kcal, protein: 30 g, carbohydrates: 7 g, Fat: 7 g, Cholesterol: 73 mg, Fiber: 0.5 g, Sodium: 88 mg, Potassium: 337 mg, Phosphorus: 230 mg, Calcium: 34 mg

### Ingredients:

- 1 tablespoon of cornstarch

- 4 skinless, boneless chicken breasts
- 1 tablespoon of olive oil
- 1/4 cup of balsamic vinegar
- 1 teaspoon of fresh ground black pepper
- 3/4 cup of sliced white button mushrooms.
- 1 bay leaf
- 3/4 cup of low-sodium chicken broth
- 1/4 teaspoon of thyme leaves
- Eight garlic cloves, peeled.

## Instructions:

Rinse chicken and cut the extra chicken breast fat. Coat the chicken breast with pepper on both ends. Heat olive oil over medium-high heat in a non-stick skillet and cook for 3 minutes or lightly browned. Add garlic, change the side of the chicken, and sprinkle mushrooms. To prevent them from sticking, turn the chicken and mushrooms and cook for around 3 minutes. Mix low-sodium chicken broth, balsamic vinegar, thyme, cornstarch, and bay leaf, in a shallow dish. Pour the mixture into a skillet. Stir until it thickens. Cover and simmer for about 10 minutes over moderately-low heat. Before serving, extract the garlic and bay leaf. Serve with rice or pasta.

## 145- Broccoli Chicken Casserole

Preparation time: 10 minutes

Cooking Time: 1 hour 20 minutes

Servings: 8

Difficulty Level: Easy

## Nutritional Information:

Calories: 287 kcal, protein: 19 g, carbohydrates: 20 g, Fat: 11 g, Cholesterol: 52 mg, Fiber: 1.8 g, Sodium: 261 mg, Potassium: 308 mg, Phosphorus: 256 mg, Calcium: 71 mg

## Ingredients:

- 1 medium onion, chopped.
- 2 cups of milk
- 2-3 cups of cooked broccoli.
- 2 eggs, beaten.
- 2-3 chicken breast, diced.
- 2 cups of grated cheese.
- 2 tablespoons of butter or margarine
- grated parmesan.
- 2 cups of cooked barley, rice, or noodles.

## Instructions:

Preheat the oven to 350°F. Put broccoli in a microwaveable dish, cover with wrap, and microwave for around 2-3 minutes until light green. And in the meantime, cook chicken and onion in butter until it turns brown on a skillet. Place all the ingredients in a greased casserole dish and mix. Sprinkle grated parmesan cheese and bake for around 1 hour and 15 mins until fully cooked.

## 146- Chicken Broccoli Stromboli

Preparation time: 10 minutes

Cooking Time: 20 minutes

Servings: 4

Difficulty Level: Medium

## Nutritional Information:

Calories: 522 kcal, protein: 38 g, carbohydrates: 52 g, Fat: 17 g, Cholesterol: 75 mg, Fiber: 2.9 g, Sodium: 607 mg, Potassium: 546 mg, Phosphorus: 400 mg, Calcium: 262 mg

## Ingredients:

- 2 tablespoons of olive oil
- 1-pound pizza dough: store-bought
- 1 cup of low-salt mozzarella cheese: shredded.
- 2 cups of broccoli florets, blanched
- 1 tablespoon of fresh garlic, chopped.

- 2 cups of chicken breast: cooked, diced.
- 1 tablespoon of fresh oregano, chopped.
- 2 tablespoons of flour
- 1 teaspoon of red pepper flakes: crushed.

## Instructions:

Preheat the oven to 400° F. In a large bowl, combine cheese, chicken, broccoli, pepper flakes, oregano, and garlic. Sprinkle flour on the workspace and spread dough to make a rectangular 11" x 14". Pour the chicken mixture along the longest line, about 2 inches from the edge of the dough. Fold and press the ends and tightly seal the edges using a fork. Brush the surface with olive oil and make 3 narrow slits. Bake on a lightly oil-greased baking sheet tray for 8 to 12 minutes or until golden brown. Takeout from the oven, allow it to set, and serve hot.

## 147- Herb-Crusted Roast Leg of Lamb

Preparation time: 10 minutes

Cooking Time: 2 hours 40 minutes

Servings: 12

Difficulty Level: Medium

### Nutritional Information:

Calories: 292 kcal, protein: 24 g, carbohydrates: 2 g, Fat: 20 g, Cholesterol: 86 mg, Fiber: 0 g, Sodium: 157 mg, Potassium: 419 mg, Phosphorus: 292 mg, Calcium: 19 mg

### Ingredients:

- Three tablespoons of lemon juice
- ½ cup of dry vermouth
- 1 leg of lamb: 4-pound
- 1 tablespoon of curry powder
- 2 cloves garlic, minced.
- 1 cup of onions, sliced.
- ½ teaspoon of ground black pepper

## Instructions:

Preheat the oven to 400° F. Put the lamb leg on a baking dish. Add 1 tsp of lemon juice; use 2 tsp of lemon juice with the remaining spices to make a paste. Marinate lamb in a paste. Roast the lamb for 30 minutes in a 400 ° F oven. Add onions and vermouth and drain off the grease. Cook at 325 ° F for 2 hours. Baste the lamb's leg occasionally. Remove from the oven when the internal temperature is 145 ° F and leave to set for 3 minutes before serving.

## 148- Herb-Roasted Chicken Breasts

Preparation time: 4 hours 10 minutes

Cooking Time: 30 minutes

Servings: 4

Difficulty Level: Medium

### Nutritional Information:

Calories: 270 kcal, protein: 26 g, carbohydrates: 3 g, Fat: 17 g, Cholesterol: 83 mg, Fiber: 0.6 g, Sodium: 53 mg, Potassium: 491 mg, Phosphorus: 252 mg, Calcium: 17 mg

### Ingredients:

- 2 tbsp of Garlic and Herb Seasoning Blend
- 1-pound of skinless, boneless chicken breasts
- 1–2 garlic cloves
- 1 medium onion
- ¼ cup of olive oil
- 1 teaspoon of black pepper: ground

### Instructions:

**To marinate:**

Slash the garlic and onion and put them in a dish. Add Seasoning, olive oil, and ground pepper. To the marinade, add chicken breasts, cover, and refrigerate it for at least 4 hours.

**For baking:**

Preheat the oven to 350°F. Put the marinated chicken breasts on foil and baking sheet lined pan. Pour over the chicken with the remaining marinade and roast for 20 minutes at 350 ° F. Bake for an extra 5 minutes for browning.

## 149- Egg Fried Rice

Preparation time: 5 minutes

Cooking Time: 10 minutes

Servings: 6

Difficulty Level: Easy

### Nutritional Information:

Calories: 343 kcal, protein: 15 g, carbohydrates: 37 g, Fat: 15 g, Cholesterol: 212 mg, Fiber: 3.2 g, Sodium: 238 mg, Potassium: 350 mg, Phosphorus: 230 mg, Calcium: 83 mg

### Ingredients:

- 1 cup of frozen peas, thawed.
- 2 teaspoons of dark sesame oil
- 1 tablespoon of canola oil
- 2 eggs
- 1 cup of bean sprouts
- 2 egg whites
- ¼ teaspoon of black pepper: ground
- 4 cups of cooked rice.
- ⅓ cup of chopped green onions.

### Instructions:

Mix the eggs, egg whites, and sesame oil in a small bowl. Stir thoroughly and put back. Warm canola oil over medium-high heat in a broad non-stick pan. Add a mixture of eggs and stir-fry until cooked. Green onions and bean sprouts are added. For 2 minutes, stir-fry. Add peas and rice. Continue to stir-fry until fully cooked. Garnish with black pepper and serve hot.

## 150- Fired-Up Zucchini Turkey Burger

Preparation time: 15 minutes

Cooking Time: 20-30 minutes

Servings: 4

Difficulty Level: Medium

### Nutritional Information:

Calories: 211 kcal, protein: 25 g, carbohydrates: 5 g, Fat: 10 g, Cholesterol: 125 mg, Fiber: 1.6 g, Sodium: 128 mg, Potassium: 475 mg, Phosphorus: 280 mg, Calcium: 43 mg

### Ingredients:

- 1 cup of shredded zucchini.
- 1 pound of ground turkey meat
- ½ cup of minced onion.
- 1 jalapeño pepper (sliced, seeded, and minced).
- 1 egg
- 2 fresh poblano peppers, sliced and seeded.
- 1 teaspoon of mustard (optional)
- 1 teaspoon of Extra Spicy Blend

### Instructions:

Thoroughly combine meat, zucchini, onion, jalapeno, egg, and spices. Create 4 turkey burger patties of meat mixture. Turkey burgers can be cooked on a grill or an electric griddle. Grill pepper along with them until the skin is blistered and tender. Grill patties until no pinkish appearance remain, at least to 165 ° F. Serve them with hamburgers.

## 151- Red Lentil Dahl

Preparation time: 10 minutes

Cooking Time: 40 minutes

Servings: 4

Difficulty Level: Medium

Calories: 230 kcal, protein: 13 g, carbohydrates: 36.5 g, Fat: 4.7 g, Cholesterol: 0 mg, Fiber: 7 g, Sodium: 104.8 mg, Potassium: 32.1 mg, Phosphorus: 169 mg, Calcium: 18 mg

## Ingredients:

- 1 Tbsp of canola oil
- 1 cup of red lentils
- 1/2 tsp of cumin powder
- 1 cup of diced yellow onion.
- 1/2 tsp cumin seeds
- 4 minced garlic cloves.
- 1 green or red chili pepper: minced.
- 1/2 tsp of ground turmeric
- 1/2 tsp paprika
- 2 Tbsp of ginger root: minced.
- 4 cherry tomatoes, quartered.
- 1/4 tsp of ground cayenne pepper
- 1 tsp of brown sugar
- Chopped cilantro leaves for garnish; Optional.
- 1/2 cup of almond milk: unsweetened
- 1 tsp of lime juice
- 1/4 tsp of black pepper: ground

## Instructions:

Dip the lentils for 12 hours or more in a big pot of water (~ 10 cups). Drain out the soaking water as it contains potassium, and rinse the lentils once done with soaking. Fill 3 cups of room temperature water in a medium pot, add the rinsed lentils and cook on medium heat for 20 minutes. Then add oil to a skillet and heat it over medium flame. Fry cumin seeds and powder for 60 to 90 seconds until aromatic. Add the chili pepper, onion, ginger, and garlic; cook for 4 to 6 minutes, or until the onions are soft. After this add the remaining spices (pepper, cayenne. turmeric, salt, paprika) and tomatoes; cook for 2 to 3 minutes or so. Pour almond milk and boil for 2 or 3 minutes more. Drain off any extra water once the lentils are cooked.

Stir in the cooked lentils with a mixture of spiced onions. Add the brown sugar and lime juice and mix well. If needed, garnish with cilantro and serve with rice.

## 152- Middle Eastern-inspired Scotch Eggs

Preparation time: 10 minutes

Cooking Time: 20 minutes

Servings: 6

Difficulty Level: Medium

## Nutritional Information:

Calories: 266 kcal, protein: 11.7 g, carbohydrates: 16.28 g, Fat: 16.71 g, Cholesterol: 157 mg, Fiber: 1 g, Sodium: 403 mg, Potassium: 162 mg, Phosphorus: 20 mg, Calcium: 60 mg

## Ingredients:

- 1 small finely chopped red onion.
- 500g of lean lamb or minced beef
- ¼ cup of pine nuts
- ¼ cup of sultanas or currants (skip if on a low potassium diet)
- 6 eggs
- ¼ cup of parsley or fresh coriander
- 2 teaspoons of sumac
- ¼ cup of plain flour
- 1 egg whisked.
- Oil for frying
- ¼ cup of dried breadcrumbs

## Instructions:

Boil six eggs until hard. Set aside 5 minutes to cool once boiled, then peel and put aside. Meanwhile, add mince, whisked egg, currants or sultanas, sumac, pine nuts, coriander or parsley, and onion in a wide bowl. Combine all the ingredients properly by hand, and make 6 equivalent parts of the mixture. In two different cups, add breadcrumbs and flour. To a flour mixture, roll peeled boiled eggs and set aside. Take 1 portion of the thin mixture in the palm of your hand and use the other palm to flatten it. Put the egg in the middle of the thin mixture. Coat the thin mixture evenly around the boiled egg.

Roll in breadcrumbs. Repeat the process for the remainder of the eggs. To a depth of around 5cm of the pan, add oil. Fry the eggs in a skillet until golden brown and place it on paper absorbent. Serve hot.

## 153- Vegetarian Reuben Sandwich

Preparation time: 15 minutes

Cooking Time: 4 minutes

Servings: 2

Difficulty Level: Easy

### Nutritional Information:

Calories: 433 kcal, protein: 12 g, carbohydrates: 31 g, Fat: 30 g, Cholesterol: 37 mg, Fiber: 4 g, Sodium: 394 mg, Potassium: 406 mg, Phosphorus: 172 mg, Calcium: 290 mg

### Ingredients:

- 2 teaspoons of olive oil
- ¼ teaspoon of coriander seeds, crushed.
- ½ teaspoon of black pepper, ground.
- 1 cornichon, chopped.
- 2 tablespoons of mayonnaise,
- 1 tablespoon of tomato paste
- ½ tablespoon of butter, unsalted, softened.
- 2 hot dog buns (6-inch x 2-inch size)
- 1 large beet
- 2 ½ tablespoons of drained and warmed sauerkraut.
- 2 slices of low sodium Swiss cheese,
- 1 tablespoon of lemon juice.

### Instructions

Boil water in a medium-sized saucepan. Add beet and lower the heat to boil until it gets tender, then cool and peel it. Cut it crosswise into ¼-inch thick slices and place them on a plate. Add 2 teaspoons olive oil to the beets, then sprinkle coriander and black pepper. To make Russian dressing, mix tomato paste, lemon juice, cornichon, and mayonnaise in a small bowl. Preheat the oven. Lengthwise, slash the buns into 2 halves and place them on a baking sheet with the cut side up. Brush over them with melted butter. For around 1 to 2 minutes, bake it. Then take them to the work surface and layer the base sides with sauerkraut, beet slices, and Russian dressings. Place a cheese slice on them and bake them for 2 minutes until the cheese melts. Cover with other halves and serve them hot.

## 154  Chicken Egg Rolls

Preparation time: 10 minutes

Cooking Time: 30 minutes

Servings: 14

Difficulty Level: Medium

### Nutritional Information:

Calories: 676 kcal, protein: 6 g, carbohydrates: 22 g, Fat: 63 g, Cholesterol: 36 mg, Fiber: 1 g, Sodium: 95 mg, Potassium: 131 mg, Phosphorus: 71 mg, Calcium: 22 mg

### Ingredients:

- 2 tablespoons of sesame oil
- 1 pound chicken thighs: diced.
- 2 cloves of minced garlic.
- ½ pound of bean sprouts: drained or 1 (14 ounces) can.
- 1 cup of chopped green onion (including the green tops).
- ½ pound of coleslaw mix

- 14 egg roll wrappers
- 1 tablespoon of low-sodium soy sauce
- ½ teaspoon of Chinese five-spice
- 2 teaspoons of minced fresh ginger.
- 3-4 cups of oil
- 2 teaspoons of sugar

## Instructions:

Mix the chicken, bean sprouts, coleslaw, onion, sesame oil, soya sauce, garlic, ginger, sugar, and spices in a bowl. Marinate for 30 minutes. As directed on the package, use 1/3 cup of filling for each wrapper and fold it. Fry it in a deep fryer or fill a frying pan with oil at least one inch deep and heat to 350 degrees F. In hot oil, fry egg rolls until golden brown. On paper towels, drain them, and serve hot.

## 155- Crab Cake

Preparation time: 10 minutes

Cooking Time: 10-15 minutes

Servings: 6

Difficulty Level: Easy

## Nutritional Information:

Calories: 188 kcal, protein: 13 g, carbohydrates: 5 g, Fat: 13 g, Cholesterol: 111 mg, Fiber: 0.5 g, Sodium: 342 mg, Potassium: 317 mg, Phosphorus: 185 mg, Calcium: 52 mg

## Ingredients:

- 1 tsp herb and spices seasoning, 30% less sodium.
- 1 pound of lump crab meat
- 1/8 tsp of cayenne pepper
- 1 slice of white bread
- 2 tbsp olive oil
- 1 tsp yellow mustard
- 1 tbsp mayonnaise
- 1 large egg
- 1 tbsp fresh parsley

## Instructions:

Hold the crab meat in a medium bowl and remove the shell parts. Slice the pieces of bread into cubes. Combine the crab with mustard, bread, mayonnaise, seasonings, minced parsley, egg, and cayenne pepper. Mix but do not over-mix until all the ingredients are combined. Portion 6 crab cakes, each 3/4" thick, using a 1/3 cup measurement. Cool it in the refrigerator for one hour. Cook for 4-5 minutes on each side until cooked. Serve warm.

## 156- Classic Pot Roast

Preparation time: 10 minutes

Cooking Time: 5 hours

Servings: 8

Difficulty Level: Medium

## Nutritional Information:

Calories: 154 kcal, protein: 13 g, carbohydrates: 3 g, Fat: 10 g, Cholesterol: 41 mg, Fiber: 0 g, Sodium: 49 mg, Potassium: 219 mg, Phosphorus: 113 mg, Calcium: 19 mg

## Ingredients:

- ½ teaspoon of black pepper: freshly ground.
- 1 pound of beef chuck or rump roast: boneless
- 1 tablespoon of olive oil
- 2 teaspoons of minced garlic
- ½ small, sweet onion: chopped.
- 1 cup of water plus 3 tablespoons of water
- 2 tablespoons of cornstarch
- 1 teaspoon of dried thyme

## Instructions:

Place a large stockpot over medium heat. Season the roast with pepper. Add the oil to the stockpot and brown the meat all over. Remove the meat to a plate; set aside. Sauté the onion and garlic in the stockpot for about 3 minutes or until they are softened. Return the beef to the pot with accumulated juices and add the thyme and 1 cup of water. Bring the liquid to a boil and then reduce the heat to low so the liquid simmers. Cover and simmer for about 4½ hours or until the beef is tender. In a small dish, stir cornstarch and 3 tablespoons of water. Add slurry to the pot with liquid and cook for 15 minutes to thicken the sauce. Serve the roast with the gravy.

## 157- Herb Rolls

Preparation time: 50 minutes

Cooking Time: 35 minutes

Servings: 18

Difficulty Level: Medium

### Nutritional Information:

Calories: 117 kcal, protein: 3 g, carbohydrates: 21 g, Fat: 8 g, Cholesterol: 0 mg, Fiber: 2 g, Sodium: 8 mg, Potassium: 75 mg, Phosphorus: 43 mg, Calcium: 15 mg

### Ingredients:

- 1 large egg, beaten.
- 3 1/2 cups of flour
- 1 package of dry yeast
- 2 tablespoons of oil
- 3 tablespoons of sugar
- 1/2 cup of milk
- 4 tablespoons of combined thyme, parsley, rosemary, chives,

### Instructions:

Stir 1/4 cup of lukewarm water with the yeast. Let it stand for 5 minutes, then add sugar. In a bowl, add the flour, create a well, and add the milk, oil, and herbs. To brush the tops, reserve 1

tablespoon of the beaten egg and add the remaining egg to the dough. Mix until combined, then knead until elastic, around 10 minutes, on a floured surface and let it rest 20-35 mins. Preheat the oven to 350°. Bake the rolls for 25-28 minutes until the tops are golden brown. Serve it warm.

## 158- Sukiyaki and rice

Preparation time: 10 minutes

Cooking Time: 15 minutes

Servings: 10

Difficulty Level: Easy

### Nutritional Information:

Calories: 495 kcal, protein: 24 g, carbohydrates: 33 g, Fat: 29 g, Cholesterol: 79 mg, Fiber: 2 g, Sodium: 161 mg, Potassium: 536 mg, Phosphorus: 251 mg, Calcium: 32 mg

### Ingredients:

- 1/2 cup of celery (cut into 1/2-inch pieces)
- 3 medium scallions (cut thin)
- 1 tablespoon of sugar
- 1 medium tomato, sliced.
- 1 tablespoon of vegetable oil
- 2 1/2 pounds of lean beef chuck
- 2 tablespoons of soy sauce: low sodium
- 1/2 cup of broccoli, frozen: chopped.
- 1 medium onion (cut into 1/8-inch slices)
- 3/4 cup of sliced mushrooms.
- 5 cups of cooked white rice.
- 1 medium green pepper (cut in rings)
- 1 tablespoon of water
- 1 cup of white turnip (cut into 1/8-inch slices)
- 1 cup of shredded cabbage

## Instructions:

Add oil to a wide heavy skillet and cook meat on both sides on both sides, until browned. Then add all vegetables into the skillet and cook them. Combine sugar, water, and soy sauce; pour it over vegetables. Cover and steam for 10-15 minutes over moderate heat. Serve with boiled rice.

# 159- Zucchini Squash Bake

Preparation time: 10 minutes

Cooking Time: 20 minutes

Servings: 4

Difficulty Level: Easy

## Nutritional Information:

Calories: 216 kcal, protein: 7 g, carbohydrates: 16 g, Fat: 14 g, Cholesterol: 129 mg, Fiber: 1.1 g, Sodium: 318 mg, Potassium: 232 mg, Phosphorus: 123 mg, Calcium: 69 mg

## Ingredients:

- 2 med. zucchini, cut into 1/4-inch slices (approximately 2 cups)
- 2 tablespoon extra-virgin olive oil
- 2 shallots, minced.
- 1.5 med. Yellow summer squash, cut into 1/4-inch slices (approximately 2 cups)
- 1/4 tsp. coarsely ground pepper
- 1/2 tsp. dried oregano
- 4 garlic cloves, minced.
- 1/2 cup grated cheddar cheese, divided.
- 1 cup panko (Japanese) breadcrumbs, divided.

## Instructions:

Preheat the oven to 450 ° F. Heat the olive oil over medium heat in a wide skillet; add the yellow squash, zucchini, and shallots. Use oregano and pepper to sprinkle. Cook and mix for 4-6 minutes until the zucchini and squash are crisp-tender. Add garlic; cook for an additional 1 minute. Then add 1/2 cup breadcrumbs and 1/4 cup cheese; remove from heat. Place it into a greased 11x7-in. Or 2-qt. Dish for baking. Sprinkle with the leftover cheese and breadcrumbs. Bake for 8-10 minutes, until golden brown.

# 160- Broiled Haddock with Cucumber Salsa

Preparation time: 10 minutes

Cooking Time: 20 minutes

Servings: 4

Difficulty Level: Medium

## Nutritional Information:

Calories: 126 kcal, protein: 22 g, carbohydrates: 6 g, Fat: 1 g, Cholesterol: 65 mg, Fiber: 0.9 g, Sodium: 80 mg, Potassium: 466 mg, Phosphorus: 232 mg, Calcium: 50 mg

## Ingredients:

- 1/2 cup of cucumber
- 1/2 teaspoon of garlic powder
- 1 small ear of fresh corn
- 1/4 cup of red onion
- 1/4 cup of red bell pepper
- 1 garlic clove
- 3 tablespoons of fresh cilantro
- 1/4 teaspoon of cayenne pepper
- 1/2 teaspoon of onion powder
- 4-1/2 tablespoons of lime juice
- 1/2 teaspoon of black pepper
- 1-pound fresh haddock

## Instructions:

Switch on the broiler. In a grill pan or hot grill, cook corn until grill marks are visible. Then remove the kernels from the stalk using a sharp knife. The cucumber is peeled and diced. Cut onion, and bell pepper into cubes, mince the garlic and chop the cilantro. Combine the onion, cucumber, red pepper, garlic clove, cilantro, cayenne pepper, 1-1/2 tbsp of lime juice, and grilled corn kernels mixing bowl. Add flavors and refrigerate them. Split fish into four fillets. Lightly cut the fillets with a fine knife. Add the pepper, onion powder, and garlic powder. Lightly drizzle the fillets with 3 tbsp of lime juice. Arrange it on a parchment-lined baking sheet. Put these sheets under the broiler and cook until cooked or golden brown. Serve with a Cucumber mixture.

# 161- Orange Chicken

Preparation time: 10 minutes

Cooking Time: 6-8 hours

Servings: 4

Difficulty Level: Easy

## Nutritional Information:

Calories: 242 kcal, protein: 14 g, carbohydrates: 19 g, Fat: 12 g, Cholesterol: 37 mg, Fiber: 0.4 g, Sodium: 340 mg, Potassium: 240 mg, Phosphorus: 118 mg, Calcium: 30 mg

## Ingredients:

- 1 Tablespoon of balsamic vinegar
- 8 bone-in chicken thighs
- ⅓ cup of flour
- 1 Tablespoon of ketchup
- medium onion, chopped.
- 4 ounces of orange juice
- medium bell pepper, chopped.
- 1 Tablespoon of brown sugar

## Instructions:

Marinate chicken with flour in a plastic bag by shaking it. To the slow cooker, add this coated chicken. Mix the brown sugar, orange juice, ketchup, and vinegar in a bowl. Pour the sauce

over the chicken into the slow cooker and mix it well. Cook for 6-8 hours, on LOW. Serve chicken with white rice and sauce.

# 162- Roasted Citrus Chicken

Preparation time: 10 minutes

Cooking Time: 6-8 hours

Servings: 4-6

Difficulty Level: Easy

## Nutritional Information:

Calories: 251 kcal, protein: 19 g, carbohydrates: 0 g, Fat: 0 g, Cholesterol: 61 mg, Fiber: 18 g, Sodium: 77 mg, Potassium: 222 mg, Phosphorus: 188 mg, Calcium: 15 mg

## Ingredients:

- 2 cloves garlic, minced.
- 1 Tablespoon of olive oil
- 2 cups chicken broth, low sodium
- 3 Tablespoons of lemon juice
- 1 teaspoon of Italian Seasoning
- ½ large chicken breast
- ½ teaspoon of black pepper

## Instructions:

In a wide skillet, heat the oil. Seasonings and garlic are added. Then add the chicken breasts and cook them on both sides. Transfer chicken breast to slow cooker and pour chicken broth in it. Cook for 6 to 8 hours on LOW heat. Add lemon juice and serve it at the end of the cooking process.

# 163- Hawaiian Chicken and Rice

Preparation time: 10 minutes

Cooking Time: 9-10 hours

Servings: 6

Difficulty Level: Easy

## Nutritional Information:

Calories: 97 kcal, protein: 2 g, carbohydrates: 20 g, Fat: 1 g, Cholesterol: 0 mg, Fiber: 1.8 g, Sodium: 135 mg, Potassium: 181 mg, Phosphorus: 67 mg, Calcium: 12 mg

## Ingredients:

- 6-inch piece of ginger, chopped.
- 1 Tablespoon of oyster-flavored sauce
- 7 cups of chicken broth: no/low sodium
- 1 Tablespoon of low sodium soy sauce
- 2 cups of white rice rinsed: uncooked.
- 1-pound of skinless, boneless chicken thighs: one-inch cubes.
- 2 medium carrots, chopped.
- Twelve medium green onions, chopped.
- Cilantro
- 1 Tablespoon of sesame oil
- 1 small green cabbage, chopped.

## Instructions:

Combine the carrots, chicken, ginger, rice, and broth in a slow cooker. Cover it and cook for 7-9 hours on LOW. Open the slow cooker and blend in the cabbage and green onions. Cook for 1 hour. Add the soy sauce, oyster sauce, sesame oil, and cilantro to the pot. Enjoy it with canned pineapple.

## 164  Rice Pilaf

Preparation time: 10 minutes

Cooking Time: 1 hour 10 minutes

Servings: 8

Difficulty Level: Easy

## Nutritional Information:

Calories: 200 kcal, protein: 2 g, carbohydrates: 35 g, Fat: 6 g, Cholesterol: 0 mg, Fiber: 1.3 g, Sodium: 147 mg, Potassium: 95 mg, Phosphorus: 47 mg, Calcium: 32 mg

## Ingredients:

- 2 Tablespoons of unsalted butter (or olive oil)
- 1-2 cloves of garlic - minced
- 1/4 cup of wild rice
- 1 cup of white rice
- Three cups of chicken stock or broth: low sodium
- 1/2 cup of chopped onions.
- 1/4 cup of orzo pasta
- 1/2 tsp of ground black pepper (optional)
- 2 Tbsp of fresh parsley (chopped fine)

## Instructions:

Preheat the oven to 350 ° F. Boil chicken stock in a saucepan. Gently sauté the onions and garlic in the butter in a frying pan until they tend to caramelize. Add the orzo and sauté until it starts to brown. Blend the rice, orzo onions, parsley, and garlic in a 1.5-2-quart casserole. Add pepper and boiling stocks carefully. Cover and bake for half an hour or until moisture is dried. Serve it warm.

## 165- Onion Pie

Preparation time: 10 minutes

Cooking Time: 40 minutes

Servings: 6

Difficulty Level: Medium

## Nutritional Information:

Calories: 218 kcal, protein: 8 g, carbohydrates: 12 g, Fat: 15 g, Cholesterol: 122 mg, Fiber: 1 g, Sodium: 420 mg, Potassium: 128 mg, Phosphorus: 184 mg, Calcium: 127 mg

## Ingredients:

- 2 Tablespoons of butter
- 1 1/2 cup of Ritz crackers, crushed.
- 2 cups of sweet Vidalia onions, sliced.

- 1/3 cup of butter, melted.
- 3/4 tsp of salt
- 2 eggs
- 1/8 tsp of black pepper
- 3/4 cup of half and half
- 1/4 cup of cheddar cheese

## Instructions:

Preheat the oven to 350 ° F. Blend 1/3 cup melted butter with Ritz crackers; press the combination securely into a 9-inch pie pan. Over medium heat, heat a medium skillet; melt 2 tablespoons of butter in a skillet and fry the onions. Don't get brown. Cook until the onions are clear, then scatter them onto the crust. Whisk the pepper, salt, half and half, and eggs in a medium dish. Spill the mixture over the onions and spread the cheese on top. Bake for 30 minutes and serve it.

## 166- Cream Cheese Pumpkin Pie

Preparation time: 1 hour 10 minutes

Cooking Time: 0 minutes

Servings: 16

Difficulty Level: Medium

### Nutritional Information:

Calories: 282 kcal, protein: 5 g, carbohydrates: 18 g, Fat: 21 g, Cholesterol: 92 mg, Fiber: 0.6 g, Sodium: 244 mg, Potassium: 130 mg, Phosphorus: 80 mg, Calcium: 57 mg

### Ingredients:

- 8 oz. of light cream cheese
- 15 oz. of pumpkin pie filling
- 2 Tbsp. cool whip per serving (for serving)
- 1 tsp of pumpkin pie spice
- 8 oz. of cool light whip
- 2 9" graham cracker pie crusts
- cinnamon

## Instructions:

Mix the cream cheese, pumpkin, and spices in a blender until well mixed. Roll softly into 8oz of the cool whip to remain soft and fluffy. Pour into pie shells. There should be a well-filled crust. For 1 hour, cover and refrigerate. To serve, cover each piece with 2 tablespoons of cool whip and garnish with cinnamon for the ideal final addition.

## 167- Saffron and Coriander Rice

Preparation time: 5 minutes

Cooking Time: 20 minutes

Servings: 4

Difficulty Level: Easy

### Nutritional Information:

Calories: 481 kcal, protein: 7 g, carbohydrates: 76 g, Fat: 16 g, Cholesterol: 38 mg, Fiber: 2 g, Sodium: 407 mg, Potassium: 149 mg, Phosphorus: 115 mg, Calcium: 51 mg

### Ingredients:

- 5 Cloves
- 100g of Basmati rice
- Pinch of saffron threads
- 2tbsp of Fresh coriander, chopped.
- 5 cardamom pods: Whole (optional)

### Instructions:

To a pan of boiling water, add the cardamom rice and cloves. Cook according to packet instructions. The rice is drained, and the whole spices are separated. Set the rice back in the pan. Whisk the rice with the saffron threads, cover, and leave for 5-10 minutes. Serve with minced coriander and desired sauces.

## 168- Taco Stuffing

Preparation time: 5 minutes

Cooking Time: 20-30 minutes

Servings: 8

Difficulty Level: Easy

## Nutritional Information:

Calories: 240 kcal, protein: 10 g, carbohydrates: 14 g, Fat: 16 g, Cholesterol: 36 mg, Fiber: 0.9 g, Sodium: 182 mg, Potassium: 214 mg, Phosphorus: 135 mg, Calcium: 85 mg

## Ingredients:

- One ¼ pound of lean beef: ground or turkey
- ½ head of shredded lettuce
- 1 teaspoon of garlic powder
- 2 tablespoons of vegetable oil
- ½ teaspoon of ground red pepper
- 1 teaspoon of Italian Seasoning
- ½ teaspoon of black pepper
- 1 teaspoon of onion powder
- ½ teaspoon of Tabasco sauce
- 1 medium of taco shells
- ½ teaspoon of nutmeg

## Instructions:

Heat oil over medium flame in a skillet and add ground meat and all ingredients except lettuce and taco shells. Cook until well mixed and meat gets tender. Fill taco shells with meat and cover with sliced lettuce.

## 169- Chicken Makhani

Preparation time: 10 minutes

Cooking Time: 40 minutes

Servings: 4

Difficulty Level: Medium

## Nutritional Information:

Calories: 214 kcal, protein: 9 g, carbohydrates: 22 g, Fat: 11 g, Cholesterol: 30 mg, Fiber: 2 g, Sodium: 51 mg, Potassium: 419 mg, Phosphorus: 130 mg, Calcium: 78 mg

## Ingredients:

### Chicken

- 2 tbsp. of oil
- 1 lb. skinless, boneless chicken thighs cut in cubes.
- Two slices ginger
- 1 onion
- 1/4 tsp. of cayenne pepper (optional)
- 1/2 cup of cilantro, chopped.
- 1/2 cup of yogurt
- 2 cups of crushed tomato: unsalted
- 1 tsp. of ground cumin
- 2 cloves of garlic
- 1 tsp. of garam masala

### Fragrant Basmati Rice

- 2 tsp. of olive oil
- 1 cup of basmati rice
- 1 cinnamon stick
- 1/2 tsp. of turmeric
- 1 bay leaf
- 1 cardamom pod
- 11/2 cup of water

## Instructions:

### Chicken

In a mixer, blend ginger, garlic, and onion to make a paste. Heat about 1 tablespoon of oil in a pan, add cumin, garam masala (optional), cayenne pepper, and paste, and cook until it turns brown. Stir in the tomatoes and simmer for 2 minutes. Add yogurt and reduce heat to a medium, boil, stirring regularly for 10 minutes. Remove and set aside from the heat. Heat one tablespoon of oil, add chicken and simmer until lightly browned. Add a few spoonsful sauces and cook until the liquid has decreased and the chicken is cooked. Stir the remaining sauce into the fried chicken and add cilantro. On low heat, cook for 5 to 10 minutes. Occasionally stir.

**Fragrant Basmati Rice**

In a saucepan, heat the oil. Slightly add spices and rice, stir it. Add water. Boil it for about 15 minutes by covering it.

# 170- Grilled Blackened Tilapia

Preparation time: 5 minutes

Cooking Time: 10 minutes

Servings: 4

Difficulty Level: Easy

## Nutritional Information:

Calories: 237 kcal, protein: 35 g, carbohydrates: 2 g, Fat: 10 g, Cholesterol: 85 mg, Fiber: 1 g, Sodium: 92 mg, Potassium: 580 mg, Phosphorus: 227.6 mg, Calcium: 37 mg

## Ingredients:

- 2 tablespoons of olive oil
- Four tilapia filets (about 6oz. each)
- 1 teaspoon of dried oregano
- Two teaspoons of smoked paprika.
- 3/4 teaspoon of cumin
- 1 teaspoon of garlic powder
- 1/2 teaspoon of cayenne pepper

## Instructions:

Ready grill over medium heat and grease it gently. Blend the Seasoning and coat the fish equally. Grill each side for about 3 minutes or until the fish flakes with a fork. Garnish with cilantro and serve with Pico de Gallo with red pepper.

# 171- Apple Pork Chops and Stuffing

Preparation time: 10 minutes

Cooking Time: 40 minutes

Servings: 6

Difficulty Level: Medium

## Nutritional Information:

Calories: 490 kcal, protein: 27 g, carbohydrates: 46 g, Fat: 22 g, Cholesterol: 57 mg, Fiber: 1 g, Sodium: 365 mg, Potassium: 410 mg, Phosphorus: 220 mg, Calcium: 26 mg

## Ingredients:

- 2 tablespoons of unsalted margarine
- For chicken; 6 ounces of lower-sodium stuffing mix
- 6 pork loin chops; boneless
- 20 ounces (1 jar/ can) apple pie filling

## Instructions:

Set the oven to 350° F. Spray cooking spray in a 9" x 13" pan. As directed on the packaging, add the stuffing mix to a bowl and stir in the margarine before setting it aside. Spread apple pie mixture on the pan's bottom. Over the apple pie filling, arrange the pork chops. Cover the pork chops with the filling. For 30 minutes, bake it while the foil is covered. Bake for 10 more minutes after removing the foil.

# 172- Dumplings Divine

Preparation time: 15 minutes

Cooking Time: 20 minutes

Servings: 6

Difficulty Level: Easy

## Nutritional Information:

Calories: 181 kcal, protein: 6 g, carbohydrates: 37 g, Fat: 1 g, Cholesterol: 2 mg, Fiber: 1.2 g, Sodium: 185 mg, Potassium: 92 mg, Phosphorus: 104 mg, Calcium: 120 mg

## Ingredients:

### Filling

- 2 Tbsp of soy sauce: low-sodium
- 1 Tbsp of finely chopped fresh ginger.
- 1/2 lbs. of ground meat (beef)
- 1 cup of cabbage, finely minced

### Dough

- 3/4 cup of water
- 2 cups of unbleached all-purpose flour

### Dipping sauce:

- 1 Tbsp of olive oil
- 1 Tbsp of balsamic vinegar
- 1 Tbsp of green onion
- toasted sesame seeds or red pepper flakes for garnish

## Instructions:

### Preparing the filling and dough

Filling: Combine the shredded cabbage, meat, soy sauce (low-sodium), and ginger in a medium dish. Put aside in a refrigerator.

Dough: Steadily add water to the flour in a separate bowl. Knee and blend until the dough is consistent and soft.

### Making Dumplings

Form 1-inch dough balls. Flatten the dough to make 3-1/2- or 4-inch diameter circles. In the middle of the circle, put around one tablespoon of filling. Get a cup of water. Drop your finger into the water to hold the wrapper together and mark the seal's exterior portion. Put the circle's opposite ends close and pinch in place. To seal

the dumpling, make pleats on either side. Boil water and move the dumplings to the pot one by one. Cook for 10-15 minutes until the meat is thoroughly cooked. Serve with sauce for dipping.

## 173- Roasted Rosemary Chicken and Vegetables

Preparation time: 10 minutes

Cooking Time: 60 minutes

Servings: 4

Difficulty Level: Medium

## Nutritional Information:

Calories: 215 kcal, protein: 30 g, carbohydrates: 8 g, Fat: 7 g, Cholesterol: 73 mg, Fiber: 3 g, Sodium: 107 mg, Potassium: 580 mg, Phosphorus: 250 mg, Calcium: 65 mg

## Ingredients:

- 1/2 bell pepper
- 1 medium carrot
- 1/2 large red onion
- 2 medium zucchinis
- 1 tablespoon of olive oil
- 8 garlic cloves
- 1/4 teaspoon of ground pepper
- 1 tablespoon of dried rosemary
- 4 chicken breasts; bone-in

## Instructions:

Set the oven to 375° F. Slice the carrot & bell pepper 1/4" thick, the zucchini 1/2" thick, the onion into 1/2" slices, and smash the garlic cloves.

In a 13" x 9" roasting pan, mix the oil, carrot, zucchini, onion, bell pepper, and garlic. Add 1/2 teaspoon of black pepper to the mixture and toss to coat. For approximately 10 minutes, roast the veggies until well cooked.

Remove the chicken breasts' skin and season the chicken with cracked black pepper and rosemary while the veggies are roasting. Once the skin has been replaced, season the chicken as desired with more pepper and rosemary.

Place the chicken, skin-side up, on top of the veggies in the roasting pan after removing it from the oven. Return to the oven and roast the chicken and veggies until they are done (about 35 minutes).

## 174 Southern Style Stuffed Peppers

Preparation time: 10 minutes

Cooking Time: 1 hour 20 minutes

Servings: 4

Difficulty Level: Medium

### Nutritional Information:

Calories: 264 kcal, protein: 20 g, carbohydrates: 28 g, Fat: 7 g, Cholesterol: 52 mg, Fiber: 2.7 g, Sodium: 213 mg, Potassium: 553 mg, Phosphorus: 209 mg, Calcium: 40 mg

### Ingredients:

- 1/2 cup of onion; chopped
- 3/4-pound ground beef
- 4 medium bell peppers
- 1-1/2 teaspoon of garlic powder
- 2 cups of cooked white rice
- 1 teaspoon of black pepper
- 3 ounces tomato sauce; unsalted
- 1 tablespoon of dried parsley

### Instructions:

Preheat an oven to 375 degrees Fahrenheit. Peppers are cored and deseeded. Drain liquid after browning ground meat. Add meat cooked to rice, garlic powder, onion, parsley, black pepper, and tomato sauce; simmer for 10 minutes. Fill the mixture inside each bell pepper. After 1 hour of baking, serve it.

## 175- Turkey and Beef Chili

Preparation time: 10 minutes

Cooking Time: 1 hour 40 minutes

Servings: 12

Difficulty Level: Medium

### Nutritional Information:

Calories: 386 kcal, protein: 27 g, carbohydrates: 38 g, Fat: 14 g, Cholesterol: 75 mg, Fiber: 2.3 g, Sodium: 300 mg, Potassium: 552 mg, Phosphorus: 278 mg, Calcium: 53 mg

### Ingredients:

- 1-pound lean beef; ground
- 2 pounds turkey; ground
- 1/2 green bell pepper
- 1 large onion,
- 1-1/2 tablespoons of cumin seed
- 1 teaspoon of salt
- 2 garlic cloves
- 1/2 teaspoon of black pepper
- 9 cups of cooked white rice
- 1 teaspoon of ground oregano
- 1/2 teaspoon of paprika
- 3 cups of boiling water
- 1 tablespoon of all-purpose white flour
- 6 ounces low sodium canned tomato paste
- 1/4 cup of chili powder

### Instructions:

Add beef and turkey to a wide skillet, and sauté it until brown. Slice the onion, green pepper, and garlic. Meat is added; stirred. Add paprika, salt, cumin, pepper, and oregano. Add flour to the mixture. Chili powder and hot water are mixed. Stir in the skillet. For one hour, cook gently. Add tomato paste and stir it thoroughly. Remove any extra oil. Cook for 30 more minutes. Over hot white rice, serve it.

## 176- Tuna Salad Bagel

Preparation time: 10 minutes

Cooking Time: 0 minutes

Servings: 1

Difficulty Level: Easy

### Nutritional Information:

Calories: 290 kcal, protein: 25 g, carbohydrates: 32 g, Fat: 7 g, Cholesterol: 22 mg, Fiber: 2.5 g, Sodium: 475 mg, Potassium: 320 mg, Phosphorus: 175 mg, Calcium: 17 mg

### Ingredients:

- 1 tablespoon of celery
- 1/2 cup of tuna; water-packed; low sodium canned
- 1 tablespoon of onion
- 1 tablespoon of mayonnaise; reduced-calorie
- 1 lettuce leaf
- 1 medium; 2-ounce bagel

### Instructions:

Break tuna into small pieces. Chop celery and onion finely. Mayonnaise, celery, onion, and tuna are mixed thoroughly. With a lettuce leaf, spread the mixture on the bagel.

## 177- BBQ Chicken Pita Pizza

Preparation time: 10 minutes

Cooking Time: 15 minutes

Servings: 2

Difficulty Level: Medium

### Nutritional Information:

Calories: 320 kcal, protein: 23 g, carbohydrates: 37 g, Fat: 9 g, Cholesterol: 55 mg, Fiber: 2.4 g, Sodium: 523 mg, Potassium: 255 mg, Phosphorus: 221 mg, Calcium: 163 mg

### Ingredients:

- 1/4 cup of purple onion
- 3 tablespoons of barbecue sauce; low-sodium
- 2 tablespoons of crumbled feta cheese
- 2 pita bread; 6-1/2" size
- 1/8 teaspoon of garlic powder
- 4 ounces chicken; cooked

### Instructions:

Set the oven to 350° F. Place two pitas on a baking pan and coat with nonstick cooking spray. Each pita should have 1 1/2 tablespoons of BBQ sauce. Spread chopped onion over pitas. Sliced chicken is placed on pitas. Sprinkle feta cheese & garlic powder on it. For 11 to 13 minutes, bake it.

## 178- Creamy Mustard Chicken

Preparation time: 10 minutes

Cooking Time: 35 minutes

Servings: 4

Difficulty Level: Medium

### Nutritional Information:

Calories: 449 kcal, protein: 30.7 g, carbohydrates: 40.8 g, Fat: 16.5 g, Cholesterol: 0 mg, Fiber: 4.8 g, Sodium: 462 mg, Potassium: 476 mg, Phosphorus: 365 mg, Calcium: 54 mg

### Ingredients:

- ½ teaspoon of garlic powder
- 4 thin-sliced chicken breasts/cutlets; (about 1 pound)
- ½ teaspoon of salt; divided
- ½ package of angel hair pasta; whole-wheat (7-8 ounces)
- ¼ cup of all-purpose flour

- ½ teaspoon of freshly ground pepper; divided
- 1 large shallot; finely chopped
- 3 tablespoons of extra-virgin olive oil; divided
- ½ cup of water
- ½ cup of dry white wine
- ¼ cup of reduced-fat sour cream
- 2 tablespoons of chopped fresh sage and more for garnish
- 2 tablespoons of Dijon mustard

## Instructions:

Bring water in a big pot to a boil. Add the pasta and prepare it as directed on the box. Drain. Meanwhile, season chicken with 1/4 teaspoon of salt, pepper, and garlic powder. Chicken is covered on both sides with flour; then, any excess should be shaken off. Only 2 tablespoons of flour are saved.

In a large skillet over medium-high heat, warm 2 tablespoons of oil. Cook the chicken for 3 to 4 minutes on each side, turning it once or until it turns golden brown and well cooked. Place on a fresh dish. Turn the heat to medium-low and pour the last tablespoon of oil into the pan. Add the shallot and stir while cooking for 30 seconds to 1 minute, or until it starts to brown. Add wine and cook for one minute while periodically stirring. Add the 2 teaspoons of flour to the water. Add to the pan and constantly whisk for 1 minute or until thickened. Remove from the heat and whisk in the remaining 1/4 teaspoon each of salt and pepper, along with the mustard, sour cream, and 2 teaspoons of sage. Turn the chicken over in the pan to evenly coat the sauce.

Pasta is placed topped with half of the sauce, followed by the chicken and the remaining sauce. If desired, add extra sage as a garnish.

## 179- Fruited Curry Chicken Salad

Preparation time: 10 minutes

Cooking Time: 0 minutes

Servings: 8

Difficulty Level: Easy

## Nutritional Information:

Calories: 238 kcal, protein: 14 g, carbohydrates: 6 g, Fat: 18 g, Cholesterol: 44 mg, Fiber: 1.1 g, Sodium: 162 mg, Potassium: 200 mg, Phosphorus: 115 mg, Calcium: 15 mg

## Ingredients:

- 1 stalk celery
- 4 cooked boneless, skinless chicken breasts
- 1/4 cup of seedless red grapes
- 1/2 cup of onion
- 1/4 cup of seedless green grapes
- 1 medium apple
- 1/8 teaspoon of black pepper
- 1/2 cup of canned water chestnuts
- 3/4 cup of mayonnaise
- 1/2 teaspoon of curry powder

## Instructions:

Chop up the chicken. Chop the apple, onion, and celery. Water chestnuts are drained and chopped. Chicken, onion, celery, curry powder, apple, grapes, pepper, water chestnuts, and mayonnaise are combined in a large salad bowl. Either serve now or chill it for later.

## 180- Sweet & Crunchy Coleslaw

Preparation time: 10 minutes

Cooking Time: 0 minutes

Servings: 12

Difficulty Level: Easy

## Nutritional Information:

Calories: 244 kcal, protein: 1 g, carbohydrates: 20 g, Fat: 19 g, Cholesterol: 0 mg, Fiber: 1 g,

Sodium: 12 mg, Potassium: 73 mg, Phosphorus: 13 mg, Calcium: 20 mg

## Ingredients:

- 1 cup of sugar
- ½ cup of sweet onion; chopped
- 1 teaspoon of celery seed
- 6 cups of shredded cabbage
- 1 cup of canola oil
- 1 teaspoon of prepared yellow mustard
- ½ cup of rice vinegar

## Instructions:

In a big bowl, combine chopped onion and cabbage. Blend the remaining ingredients in a blender until fully blended. Over the onion and cabbage, pour the dressing. Stir well, then refrigerate it. Serve it

## 181- Hawaiian-Style Pulled Pork

Preparation time: 10 minutes

Cooking Time: 4-5 hours

Servings: 16

Difficulty Level: Medium

## Nutritional Information:

Calories: 285 kcal, protein: 20 g, carbohydrates: 1 g, Fat: 21 g, Cholesterol: 83 mg, Fiber: 0 g, Sodium: 54 mg, Potassium: 380 mg, Phosphorus: 230 mg, Calcium: 9 mg

## Ingredients:

- ½ teaspoon of paprika
- 4 pounds of pork roast
- ½ teaspoon of ground black pepper
- 1 teaspoon of onion powder
- 2 tablespoons of liquid smoke
- ½ teaspoon of garlic powder

- Optional garnish: (radishes or pickled red onions) 1 red onion /4 radishes, ⅓ cup of white vinegar & ¼ teaspoon of sugar

## Instructions:

Mix the black pepper, paprika, onion, and garlic powder in a small bowl. The pork should be rubbed with the spice mixture all over. Put the pork in a crockpot or slow cooker, and add some liquid smoke. Fill slow cooker or crockpot with water until it measures 1/4–1/2" deep. Cook for 4-5 hours on high. Using two forks, remove the pork from the cooking liquid, then shred the flesh. Sliced radishes or pickled red onions are used as a garnish.

## 182- Mediterranean Green Beans

Preparation time: 5 minutes

Cooking Time: 10 minutes

Servings: 4

Difficulty Level: Easy

## Nutritional Information:

Calories: 71 kcal, protein: 2 g, carbohydrates: 10 g, Fat: 3 g, Cholesterol: 0 mg, Fiber: 3.7 g, Sodium: 2 mg, Potassium: 186 mg, Phosphorus: 37 mg, Calcium: 55 mg

## Ingredients:

- ¾ cup of water
- 3 tablespoons of fresh lemon juice
- 1-pound fresh green beans; 1- to 2-inch pieces
- 2 ½ teaspoons of olive oil
- 1/8 teaspoon of ground black pepper
- 3 fresh garlic cloves; minced

## Instructions:

In a large nonstick pan, bring the water to a boil. Add the beans, simmer for 3 minutes, then drain and put aside. Add oil to a pan that has been heated over medium-high heat. After one minute, add the beans and garlic. Add the juice & pepper and cook for 1 minute. Serve it warm.

## 183- Pumpkin Strudel

Preparation time: 25 minutes

Cooking Time: 20 minutes

Servings: 8

Difficulty Level: Medium

### Nutritional Information:

Calories: 180 kcal, protein: 3 g, carbohydrates: 25 g, Fat: 8 g, Cholesterol: 16 mg, Fiber: 2.0 g, Sodium: 141 mg, Potassium: 119 mg, Phosphorus: 39 mg, Calcium: 19 mg

### Ingredients:

- ⅛ teaspoon of grated nutmeg
- 4 tablespoons of sugar
- 1½ cups of canned pumpkin, unsweetened, sodium-free,
- 1 teaspoon of pure vanilla extract
- ½ teaspoon of ground cinnamon
- 12 sheets of phyllo dough (for defrosting, follow package directions if frozen)
- ½ stick butter (4 tablespoons), melted, unsalted,

### Instructions:

Set the oven rack in the center of the oven. Set an oven to 375° F. The canned pumpkin, vanilla essence, nutmeg, 2 tbsps. of sugar, & 1/2 tsps of cinnamon are mixed well in a medium-sized bowl.

Melted butter is applied with a pastry brush to the bottom of the medium nonstick sheet pan. One sheet of phyllo dough is placed on a spotless work surface, and butter is brushed over it. After that, stack the buttered phyllo sheets by applying butter to each one. (Remember to save enough melted butter from

coating the top of filled strudel wrapped up; use caution while brushing between layers.) To prevent them from drying out, keep the leftover phyllo dough sheets wrapped in plastic until you're ready to use them.

Spoon the mixture equally along one stack's long edges once all 12 sheets have been used. With the seam-side facing down, roll from filled end to unfilled end. Place the roll seam-side on the oiled sheet tray and brush with the remaining butter.

Mix remaining cinnamon and sugar in a small bowl. Sprinkle it on the strudel's top and sides. Bake on the center rack for 12 to 15 minutes, or until gently toasted and golden brown. Let it rest for 5 to 10 minutes after removing it from the oven before being cut with a sharp knife to enable the center to set. Serve it.

## 184- Baked Potato Soup

Preparation time: 5 minutes

Cooking Time: 20-30 minutes

Servings: 6

Difficulty Level: Medium

### Nutritional Information:

Calories: 216 kcal, protein: 15 g, carbohydrates: 29 g, Fat: 1 g, Cholesterol: 29.2 mg, Fiber: 4 g, Sodium: 272 mg, Potassium: 594 mg, Phosphorus: 326 mg, Calcium: 171.6 mg

### Ingredients:

- 1/3 cup of flour
- 2 large potatoes
- 1/2 cup of sour cream; fat-free
- 4 cups of skim milk
- 4 ounces; reduce fat shredded Monterey jack cheese
- 1/2 teaspoon of pepper

## Instructions:

Potatoes should be fork-tender after baking at 400 degrees F. Cool down. Scoop out pulp after making a longitudinal cut. Add flour to a big saucepan. Add the milk gradually while whisking to combine. Pepper and potato pulp is added. Stirring regularly, cook the food over medium heat until it thickens and bubbles. Add the cheese and stir until it melts. Sour cream is added after the heat is turned off.

## 185- Chipotle Wings

Preparation time: 5 minutes

Cooking Time: 20 minutes

Servings: 4

Difficulty Level: Easy

### Nutritional Information:

Calories: 384 kcal, protein: 20 g, carbohydrates: 18 g, Fat: 26 g, Cholesterol: 156 mg, Fiber: 0 g, Sodium: 99 mg, Potassium: 266 mg, Phosphorus: 146 mg, Calcium: 21 mg

### Ingredients:

- ¼ cup of honey
- 1-pound of fresh jumbo chicken wings; 20 individual pieces
- 1½ tablespoons of diced chipotle peppers in the adobo sauce*
- Oil; for greasing the baking sheet tray
- ¼ cup of unsalted butter; slightly melted
- 1 tablespoon of chopped chives
- 1 teaspoon of black pepper
- Cans of chipotle peppers in an adobo sauce may be found in most grocers' Latino/Mexican/ethnic cuisine.

### Instructions:

Set the oven to 400° F. On a large, oiled nonstick baking sheet pan, arrange the precut wings.

Bake for 18 to 20 minutes, flipping once, or until golden brown and an instant-read thermometer reads 165 degrees Fahrenheit. Blend the remaining ingredients in a large bowl with a rubber spatula until evenly combined. After taking the wings out of the oven, slather them with sauce. Serve after being transferred to a wide plate.

## 186- Beef or Chicken Enchiladas

Preparation time: 10 minutes

Cooking Time: 30- 40 minutes

Servings: 6

Difficulty Level: Medium

### Nutritional Information:

Calories: 235 kcal, protein: 13 g, carbohydrates: 30 g, Fat: 9 g, Cholesterol: 30 mg, Fiber: 14 g, Sodium: 201 mg, Potassium: 222 mg, Phosphorus: 146 mg, Calcium: 49 mg

### Ingredients:

- 1/2 cup of onion; chopped
- 1-pound ground lean beef or chicken
- 1/2 teaspoon of black pepper
- 1 teaspoon of cumin
- 1 garlic clove; chopped
- 1 can of enchilada sauce
- 12 corn tortillas

### Instructions:

Preheat an oven to 375-degree F. In the cooking pan, cook the meat until browned. Add the pepper, cumin, onion, and garlic. Cook it. Until the onions are tender, stir. In another skillet, heat a little oil and cook the tortillas. Put some enchilada sauce on each tortilla. Roll up after filling with meat mixture. Put the enchilada in a shallow dish/pan and, if like, cover with sauce and cheese. Enchiladas are baked until the cheese is golden and melted. Serve with your choice of topping, such as sour cream/ chopped olives.

## 187- Dilled Fish

Preparation time: 5 minutes

Cooking Time: 20 minutes

Servings: 6

Difficulty Level: Easy

### Nutritional Information:

Calories: 112 kcal, protein: 23 g, carbohydrates: 1 g, Fat: 0 g, Cholesterol: 49 mg, Fiber: 0 g, Sodium: 63 mg, Potassium: 350 mg, Phosphorus: 194 mg, Calcium: 9 mg

### Ingredients:

- 1 teaspoon of instant onion; (freeze-dried), minced
- 1 1/2 pounds fresh and firm white fish
- 1/4 teaspoon of mustard powder
- Dash of pepper
- 1/2 teaspoon of dill weed
- 4 teaspoons of lemon juice

### Instructions:

Set oven to 475 degrees Fahrenheit. Dry off the fish after rinsing it. Place in baking pan. In 2 tablespoons of water, combine mustard, onion, dill weed, & pepper. Pour lemon juice over the fish after mixing the spice with it. Bake for 17 to 20 minutes uncovered. Serve warm.

## 188- Fruit Vinegar Chicken

Preparation time: 25 minutes

Cooking Time: 30 minutes

Servings: 6

Difficulty Level: Easy

### Nutritional Information:

Calories: 413 kcal, protein: 28 g, carbohydrates: 3 g, Fat: 9.6 g, Cholesterol: 91 mg, Fiber: 6 g, Sodium: 106 mg, Potassium: 335 mg, Phosphorus: 227 mg, Calcium: 17 mg

### Ingredients:

- 1/2 cup of fruit/berry vinegar
- 1/2 teaspoon of basil
- 2 pounds chicken
- 1/2 teaspoon of tarragon
- 1/4 cup of oil
- 1/2 teaspoon of marjoram
- 1/4 cup of orange juice

### Instructions:

Preheat an oven to 350 degrees Fahrenheit. All ingredients are well combined in a big zip lock bag. Refrigerate for 15 to 20 minutes to marinate. Put the chicken on a baking dish after removing it from the bag. Bake the chicken for approximately 30 minutes, or until it reaches a temperature of about165 degrees F inside.

## 189- Chicken Lettuce Wraps

Preparation time: 15 minutes

Cooking Time: 15 minutes

Servings: 2

Difficulty Level: Easy

### Nutritional Information:

Calories: 246 kcal, protein: 33.5 g, carbohydrates: 5.8 g, Fat: 9.2 g, Cholesterol: 10.3 mg, Fiber: 1.5 g, Sodium: 154 mg, Potassium: 258.4 mg, Phosphorus: 127 mg, Calcium: 20 mg

### Ingredients:

**For Chicken:**

- 1 tablespoon avocado oil

- ½ small onion, chopped finely.
- ½ teaspoon fresh ginger, minced.
- 1 garlic clove, minced.
- ½ pound ground chicken
- Salt and freshly ground black pepper, to taste.

**For Wraps:**

- 5 romaine lettuce leaves
- 1/2 cup carrot peeled and julienned.
- ½ tablespoons fresh parsley, chopped finely.
- ½ tablespoon fresh lime juice

## Instructions:

Heat the oil over medium heat in a skillet and sauté the onion, ginger, and garlic for about 4-5 minutes. Add the ground chicken, salt, and black pepper, and cook over medium-high heat for about 7-9 minutes, breaking the meat into smaller pieces with a wooden spoon. Remove from the heat and set aside to cool. Arrange the lettuce leaves onto serving plates. Place the cooked chicken over each lettuce leaf and top with carrot and cilantro. Drizzle with lime juice and serve it.

## 190- Peas Rice

Preparation time: 5 minutes

Cooking Time: 30 minutes

Servings: 2

Difficulty Level: Easy

## Nutritional Information:

Calories: 407 kcal, protein: 8.3 g, carbohydrates: 78.8 g, Fat: 7.1 g, Cholesterol: 5 mg, Fiber: 2.9 g, Sodium: 45 mg, Potassium: 65.5 mg, Phosphorus: 12 mg, Calcium: 25 mg

## Ingredients:

- 2 whole cloves
- 1 cup of basmati rice
- ¼ teaspoon of white sugar
- 1 (2 inches) piece of cinnamon stick
- 2 cups of water
- 1 tablespoon of margarine or butter
- ¼ cup of green peas
- 1 chopped serrano pepper,
- salt to taste
- 1 teaspoon of fresh minced ginger root

## Instructions:

Rice should be washed and drained. Over medium heat, heat a saucepan. Allow the butter or margarine to melt. Add the Serrano chili, cinnamon, cloves, and ginger, and mix well. Cook for a few minutes. Stir in the rice to evenly coat it. Add salt, peas, and sugar. Fill the pan with water and boil it. Reduce the heat to a low simmer and cook the rice for 15 to 20 minutes, or until it is soft.

# CHAPTER 8

## Dinner Recipes

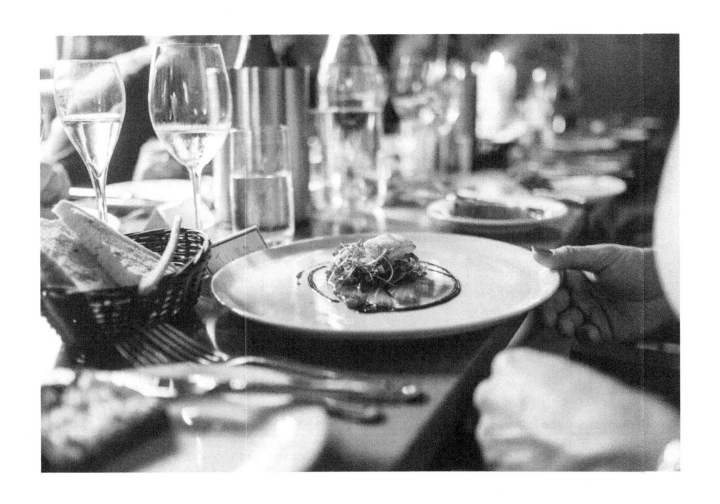

## 191- Chicken with Mustard Sauce

Preparation time: 5 minutes

Cooking Time: 25 minutes

Servings: 8

Difficulty Level: Easy

### Nutritional Information:

Calories: 361 kcal, protein: 28 g, carbohydrates: 9 g, Fat: 23 g, Cholesterol: 98 mg, Fiber: 0.6 g, Sodium: 300 mg, Potassium: 471 mg, Phosphorus: 278 mg, Calcium: 17 mg

### Ingredients:

- ¼ cup of diced shallots.
- 2 pounds of chicken breast: thinly sliced.
- ¼ cup of fresh scallions, chopped.
- ½ cup of flour
- 2 cups of low-sodium chicken stock
- ½ cup of canola oil
- 2 tablespoons of brown mustard
- 1 tablespoon of Chicken Base (low sodium)
- ½ stick of unsalted butter, cubed.
- 1 tablespoon of smoked paprika.
- 1 tablespoon of dried parsley
- ½ teaspoon of black pepper
- ½ teaspoon of Italian seasoning

### Instructions:

In a small dish, blend the Italian seasoning, pepper, parsley, and paprika. Coat the chicken breast with half of this dry blend and add the rest to the flour. Heat oil over medium-high heat in a large skillet. Set aside 3 tablespoons of seasoned flour, coat chicken in seasoned flour, then sauté both sides for 2 to 3 minutes in oil.

Remove the chicken and put it aside to rest on a plate. Take out a few tablespoons of oil and add shallots, sauté till mildly translucent. Stir until smooth, and add stock while stirring. Reduce heat and add unsalted butter, mustard, and

chicken bouillon after 5 minutes of cooking over medium-high heat. Remove from heat and return all juice drippings and the chicken to the pan from the plate and stir. Serve with scallions.

## 192- Pesto-Crusted Catfish

Preparation time: 20 minutes

Cooking Time: 20 minutes

Servings: 6

Difficulty Level: Easy

### Nutritional Information:

Calories: 312 kcal, protein: 26 g, carbohydrates: 15 g, Fat: 16 g, Cholesterol: 83 mg, Fiber: 0.8 g, Sodium: 272 mg, Potassium: 576 mg, Phosphorus: 417 mg, Calcium: 80 mg

### Ingredients:

- ½ teaspoon of black pepper
- 2 pounds of catfish (boned and filleted) 6 5-ounce pieces
- ¾ cup panko breadcrumbs
- 4 teaspoons of pesto
- ½ cup of mozzarella cheese
- 2 tablespoons of olive oil
- ½ teaspoon of dried oregano
- 1 teaspoon of garlic powder
- ½ teaspoon of red pepper flakes
- 1 teaspoon of onion powder

### Instructions:

Preheat the oven to 400° F. In a small bowl, mix all the seasonings and coat them evenly on both sides of the fish. Cover fillets with pesto and put them aside. Mix the breadcrumbs, cheese, and oil in a medium bowl and wrap the fish in this mixture well. Oil baking sheet tray and lay pesto fish on a tray with fillet side up.

Bake on the bottom rack for 15-20 minutes at 400 ° F or until brown. After cooking, leave to rest for 10 minutes and remove from the tray to avoid breaking the fish. Serve hot.

## 193- Baked Meatloaf

Preparation time: 15 minutes

Cooking Time: 25 minutes

Servings: 6

Difficulty Level: Medium

### Nutritional Information:

Calories: 205 kcal, protein: 17 g, carbohydrates: 14 g, Fat:9 g, Cholesterol: 81 mg, Fiber: 0.4 g, Sodium: 263 mg, Potassium: 254 mg, Phosphorus: 147 mg, Calcium: 36 mg

### Ingredients:

- 2 tablespoons of mayonnaise
- 1 egg, beaten.
- 1 pound of 85% ground turkey or lean ground beef
- ½ cup of panko breadcrumbs
- 1 teaspoon of garlic powder
- 1 teaspoon of Beef Base (low sodium)
- 1 teaspoon of onion powder
- ½ teaspoon of red pepper flakes
- 1 tablespoon of Worcestershire sauce: low-sodium

### Instructions:

Preheat the oven to 375 ° F. In a medium-size dish, combine all ingredients except ground turkey or beef and mix thoroughly, then add ground meat. Place the mixture in a meatloaf on a wide baking sheet-covered tray/pan. Cover and bake with aluminum foil for 20 minutes, lift the foil and cook for an extra 5 minutes. Switch off the oven and leave it to rest in the oven before serving for 10 minutes at least.

## 194- Chicken and Gnocchi Dumplings

Preparation time: 10 minutes

Cooking Time: 45 minutes

Servings: 10

Difficulty Level: Medium

### Nutritional Information:

Calories: 362 kcal, protein: 28 g, carbohydrates: 38 g, Fat: 10 g, Cholesterol: 58 mg, Fiber: 2 g, Sodium: 121 mg, Potassium: 485 mg, Phosphorus: 295 mg, Calcium: 38 mg

### Ingredients:

- 1 teaspoon of Italian seasoning
- 2 pounds of chicken breast
- ¼ cup of grapeseed or light olive oil
- 1-pound of gnocchi (store-bought)
- Six cups of chicken stock: reduced-sodium.
- ½ cup of fresh carrots: finely diced.
- 1 tablespoon of Chicken Base (low sodium)
- ½ cup of celery: fresh, finely diced.
- One teaspoon of black pepper
- ¼ cup of fresh parsley, chopped.
- ½ cup of fresh onions, finely diced.

### Instructions:

Add oil to a stockpot and place it over a high flame burner. Add chicken and cook until golden brown on both sides. Then add onions, carrots, celery, and chicken stock and cook for 20 to 30 minutes on high heat. Add black pepper, Italian seasoning, and chicken bouillon and stir on low heat. Then add gnocchi and cook, continuously stirring for 15 minutes. Remove from heat and garnish with parsley.

## 195- Chicken Pot Pie Stew

Preparation time: 10 minutes

Cooking Time: 60 minutes

Servings: 8

Difficulty Level: Medium

## Nutritional Information:

Calories: 335 kcal, protein: 32 g, carbohydrates: 42 g, Fat: 4 g, Cholesterol: 70 mg, Fiber: 3.3 g, Sodium: 118 mg, Potassium: 521 mg, Phosphorus: 290 mg, Calcium: 59 mg

## Ingredients:

- 1 cup of Cheddar cheese: low-fat
- 1½ pounds of chicken breast (boneless, skinless)
- ¼ cup of canola oil
- 2 cups of chicken stock: low-sodium
- ½ cup of carrots, diced.
- ¼ cup of celery, diced.
- 1 tablespoon of Italian seasoning: sodium-free
- 2 teaspoons of Chicken Base (low sodium)
- ½ cup of flour
- ½ cup of sweet peas, thawed.
- ½ cup of fresh onions, diced.
- 1 frozen cooked pie crust: bite-size pieces.
- ½ cup of heavy cream
- ½ teaspoon of black pepper

## Instructions:

Tenderize a pound of chicken and split it into small cubes. Put the stock and chicken in a wide stockpot and cook for 30 minutes on medium-high heat. Meanwhile, combine flour and oil until well mixed. Then add it into the mixture of chicken broth and stir until thickened. For 15 minutes, reduce the heat to medium-low and add the Italian seasoning, onions, carrots, bouillon, black pepper, and celery. For an extra 15 minutes, cook it. Remove from heat and add cream and peas. Whisk until well combined. Garnish with cheese and piecrust; serve in mugs.

## 196- Skirt Steak

Preparation time: 60 minutes

Cooking Time: 40 minutes

Servings: 4

Difficulty Level: Medium

## Nutritional Information:

Calories: 456 kcal, protein: 48.7 g, carbohydrates: 0 g, Fat: 29.1 g, Cholesterol: 168.3 mg, Fiber: 0 g, Sodium: 119 mg, Potassium: 482.2 mg, Phosphorus: 334.9 mg, Calcium: 13.6 mg

## Ingredients:

**Sauce:**

- 2 tablespoons of Dijon mustard
- ¼ cup of diced shallots.
- 1 cup of apple cider
- 1 tablespoon of black pepper
- 3 tablespoons of butter: unsalted, cubed, and chilled
- ¼ cup of dark brown sugar

**Skirt Steak:**

- ½ teaspoon of dried oregano
- 2 pounds of skirt steak
- 1 teaspoon of black pepper
- 2 tablespoons of grapeseed oil
- 1 tablespoon of vinegar
- ½ teaspoon of smoked paprika.

## Instructions:

**Bourbon Glaze:**

On a medium-high flame, cook shallots in 1 tablespoon of butter in a shallow saucepan. Lower the heat to medium, remove the pan from the burner, add bourbon, and place it back on the burner. Cook until reduced to one-third; for 10-15 minutes. Add black pepper, brown sugar, and mustard to the mixture and whisk. Remove from heat and whisk in the remaining cubed butter, almost 2 tablespoons; stir until well mixed.

**Skirt Steak:**

In a gallon-sized sealable bag, combine all ingredients, add steaks, and mix well. Let them marinate in a bag for 30-45 minutes at room temperature. Take out steaks from the bag, grill both sides for 15-20 minutes, then remove and leave to sit for 10 minutes. Slice them and serve with sauce.

# 197- Sauce-less BBQ Back Ribs

Preparation time: 20 minutes

Cooking Time: 2 hours 15 minutes

Servings: 12

Difficulty Level: Medium

## Nutritional Information:

Calories: 324 kcal, protein: 18 g, carbohydrates: 33 g, Fat: 15 g, Cholesterol: 58 mg, Fiber: 2.3 g, Sodium: 102 mg, Potassium: 453 mg, Phosphorus: 198 mg, Calcium: 47 mg

## Ingredients:

- 12 fresh or frozen mini-ears, corn cob,
- 2 slabs of baby back ribs: (about 3½ pounds)
- 1 portion of the rub
- 2 teaspoons of dark chili powder
- 1 cup of dark brown sugar.
- 1 teaspoon of black pepper
- 2 teaspoons of dehydrated onion flakes
- 1 teaspoon of red pepper flakes
- 1 teaspoon of smoked paprika.

## Instructions:

Preheat the oven to 400° F. Coat all slabs of ribs with rub mixture on both sides. Position the ribs in a rack-lined wire tray. Cover the aluminum foil securely and bake for 2 hours. Take it out from the oven and remove the foil. Set the ribs aside using tongs. Drain the liquid and bring the ribs back on the tray. Cook for 15 minutes or until the perfect crispness is achieved. Leave for 5 to 10 minutes to set, then cut and eat.

**Option to prepare on the grill:**

To avoid burning, indirect cooking in a barbecue pit is advised. For the first 3 hours, cook the ribs at 250 ° F (curled side of ribs facing up) and then raise the temperature for the last 3 hours to 300 ° F. Cover the corn in aluminum foil and put it on the grill for around 25 minutes until the maize is soft, turning periodically.

# 198- Chili Cornbread Casserole

Preparation time: 10 minutes

Cooking Time: 55 minutes

Servings: 8

Difficulty Level: Medium

## Nutritional Information:

Calories: 392 kcal, protein: 17 g, carbohydrates: 33 g, Fat: 21 g, Cholesterol: 74 mg, Fiber: 2.9 g, Sodium: 335 mg, Potassium: 441 mg, Phosphorus: 239 mg, Calcium: 156 mg

## Ingredients:

**Chili:**

- 2 tablespoons of chopped jalapeño peppers.
- 1 pound of ground beef
- and ½ cup of chopped red or green peppers.
- ½ cup of onions, diced.
- 1 tablespoon of chili powder
- ¼ cup of celery, diced.
- 1 tablespoon of garlic powder: granulated

- 1 tablespoon of cumin
- 2 tablespoons of dried onion flakes
- ½ cup of tomato sauce, no salt
- 1 teaspoon of ground black pepper
- ¼ cup of Worcestershire sauce, low-sodium
- ¼ cup of water
- 1 cup of shredded cheddar cheese.
- 1 cup of kidney beans (rinsed and drained).

**Cornbread:**

- ¾ cup of milk
- ¼ cup of cornmeal
- ¼ teaspoon of baking soda
- ¾ cup of flour
- ½ cup of sugar
- 1 egg, beaten.
- ½ teaspoon of cream of tartar
- ¼ cup of canola oil
- 1½ tablespoons of butter, unsalted, melted.

## Instructions:

Brown ground beef in a wide saucepan with jalapeños, bell peppers, celery, and onions. Drain extra oil. Then add the garlic powder, chili powder, onion flakes, tomato sauce, cumin, black pepper, water, beans, and Worcestershire sauce. For an extra 10 minutes, cook. Remove from heat and put into a baking pan measuring 9" x 9" and then garnish with cheese. Mix the baking soda, cornmeal, tartar cream, sugar, and flour, in a medium-sized dish.

Place the egg, oil, milk, and melted butter, in a small cup and mix it. Fold together the flour mixture and the egg mixture. Add the mixture over chili and bake uncovered for 25 minutes, then covered at 350 ° F for 20 minutes, taken out from the oven, and allowed to rest for 5 minutes.

# 199- Spaghetti and Asparagus Carbonara

Preparation time: 5 minutes

Cooking Time: 15 minutes

Servings: 6

Difficulty Level: Easy

## Nutritional Information:

Calories: 304 kcal, protein: 9 g, carbohydrates: 27 g, Fat: 19 g, Cholesterol: 78 mg, Fiber: 5.4 g, Sodium: 141 mg, Potassium: 287 mg, Phosphorus: 143 mg, Calcium: 95 mg

## Ingredients:

- 3 tablespoons of Parmesan cheese: shredded
- 2 teaspoons of canola oil
- 3 tablespoons of bacon bits (meatless)
- 1 cup of diced fresh onions.
- ¼ cup of chicken stock: low-sodium
- 1 large beaten egg.
- 3 cups spiral noodle pasta: cooked, cooked al dente (about 1 ½ cups raw)
- 1 cup of heavy cream
- 1 teaspoon of coarse black pepper: freshly cracked.
- 2 cups of chopped fresh asparagus (about 1" long pieces)
- ½ cup of fresh scallions, chopped.

## Instructions:

Heat the oil and cook onions in a large non-stick pan over medium-high heat until lightly browned. Meanwhile, mix the cream and the egg in a small bowl until combined. Lower the heat and pour the mixture of cream onto the onions; stir continuously for around 4 to 6 minutes with a wooden spoon until it thickens. Add the pasta, stock, black pepper, and asparagus and mix for another 3-4 minutes or until thoroughly warmed. Remove from heat and put it into a serving dish with the carbonara.

Cover and serve with cheese, scallions, and bacon bits.

## 200- Slow-Cooked Lemon Chicken

Preparation time: 10 minutes

Cooking Time: 3 hours 20 minutes

Servings: 4

Difficulty Level: Medium

### Nutritional Information:

Calories: 197 kcal, protein: 26 g, carbohydrates: 1 g, Fat: 9 g, Cholesterol: 99 mg, Fiber: 0.3 g, Sodium: 57 mg, Potassium: 412 mg, Phosphorus: 251 mg, Calcium: 20 mg

### Ingredients:

- 2 minced cloves garlic.
- 1 teaspoon of dried oregano
- 2 tablespoons of butter, unsalted
- ¼ teaspoon of ground black pepper
- 1 teaspoon of fresh basil, chopped.
- ¼ cup of low sodium chicken broth,
- 1 pound of chicken breast, skinless, boneless,
- 1 tablespoon of lemon juice
- ¼ cup of water

### Instructions:

In a small bowl, mix the ground black pepper and oregano. Coat mixture on the chicken. Then, melt the butter into a medium-size pan, brown the chicken over medium heat, and shift the chicken to the slow cooker.

Add water, chicken broth, garlic, and lemon to the skillet. Boil it, so the browned pieces are loosened, and pour it over the chicken. Cover it and set the slow cooker low for 2 1/2 hours or 5 hours. Sprinkle basil and baste the chicken. Cover and cook for 15-30 minutes or until the chicken is tender.

## 201- Spicy Beef Stir-Fry

Preparation time: 25 minutes

Cooking Time: 30 minutes

Servings: 6

Difficulty Level: Medium

### Nutritional Information:

Calories: 352 kcal, protein: 25 g, carbohydrates: 27 g, Fat: 16 g, Cholesterol: 54 mg, Fiber: 0.9 g, Sodium: 172 mg, Potassium: 390 mg, Phosphorus: 258 mg, Calcium: 32 mg

### Ingredients:

- 1 large beaten egg.
- 2 Tablespoons of cornstarch, separated.
- ¼ teaspoon of sesame oil
- 1 cup sliced onions.
- ½ teaspoon of sugar
- 2 Tablespoons of water, separated.
- 3 Tablespoons of canola oil, separated.
- One sliced green bell pepper.
- 12 ounces of the sliced beef round tip.
- 1 tablespoon of sherry
- ¼ teaspoon of red chili pepper: ground (or to taste)
- Optional garnish: parsley
- 2 teaspoons of soy sauce, low-sodium

### Instructions:

Whisk one tablespoon of water, one tablespoon of cornstarch,1 egg, and one tablespoon of canola oil in a large bowl, then add beef. For 20 minutes, marinate it. Combine the remaining water and cornstarch in a separate bowl. Put aside. Heat a skillet with the remaining 2 tablespoons of canola oil and add the meat mixture. Cook until the browning of the meat begins. Add the chili pepper, green bell peppers, sherry, and onion. Then stir-fry everything for 1 minute. Add soy-sesame oil, sauce, and sugar.

Add cornstarch and water mixture to make it thick. Cook until done. Serve hot.

# 202- Bacon, Egg, and Shrimp Grit Cakes & Smoky Cheese Sauce

Preparation time: 10 minutes

Cooking Time: 60 minutes

Servings: 6

Difficulty Level: Medium

## Nutritional Information:

Calories: 390 kcal, protein: 15 g, carbohydrates: 20 g, Fat: 28 g, Cholesterol: 170 mg, Fiber: 1.1 g, Sodium: 831 mg, Potassium: 230 mg, Phosphorus: 240 mg, Calcium: 154 mg

## Ingredients:

- 3 tablespoons of flour
- 4 eggs, beaten.
- ½ cup of onions, diced.
- 2 tablespoons of butter, unsalted
- 12 raw, peeled, deveined, and chopped shrimp.
- Four slices of bacon, low sodium: cubed.
- ½ cup of chicken stock, no salt
- 1 teaspoon of low sodium Seasoning
- 2 teaspoons of chicken flavor base, reduced-sodium.
- ¼ cup of chives, chopped.
- 1 cup milk (½ cup for the grits and ½ cup for the sauce)
- 2 tablespoons of canola oil
- ½ cup of grits
- ½ teaspoon of smoked paprika.
- ¼ cup of shredded cheddar cheese.
- ½ teaspoon of ground black pepper
- ¼ cup of Monterey Jack, Havarti, or provolone cheese
- ¼ cup of canola oil

## Instructions:

In a broad non-stick cooking pan, heat canola oil and scramble the eggs until cooked, but do not dry them. Then transfer cooked eggs to a medium-sized dish and put them aside. Now sauté the bacon, onions, shrimp, half of the chives, and seasonings in butter until the shrimp is softly yellow. Place them in the same dish as the eggs. Add bouillon, chicken broth, grits, and milk, to the same pan and cook according to packet instructions. Turn the heat off and add the mixture of egg, shrimp, and bacon into grits. Then place the mixture into a 9" x 9" baking pan that is lightly oiled and spread it evenly, then cover and refrigerate until it gets firm, and then cut it into 6 pieces.

Heat the milk (for sauce) in a saucepan, then whisk in the black pepper, cheese, the remaining chives, and paprika. Heat canola oil in a wide frying pan. Dust the grit cakes gently with flour and stir-fry until golden brown. Serve with smoky cheese sauce.

# 203- Sautéed Collard Greens

Preparation time: 5 minutes

Cooking Time: 15 minutes

Servings: 6

Difficulty Level: Easy

## Nutritional Information:

Calories: 79 kcal, protein: 2 g, carbohydrates: 4 g, Fat: 7 g, Cholesterol: 5 mg, Fiber: 2.2 g, Sodium: 9 mg, Potassium: 129 mg, Phosphorus: 18 mg, Calcium: 118 mg

## Ingredients:

- 1 tablespoon of butter, unsalted
- 8 cups of collard greens: chopped and blanched.
- 1 tablespoon of fresh garlic, chopped.
- 2 tablespoons of olive oil

- 1 teaspoon of red pepper flakes: crushed.
- ¼ cup of onions, finely diced.
- 1 tablespoon of vinegar (optional)
- 1 teaspoon of ground black pepper

## Instructions:

Cook the collard greens by placing them for 30 seconds in a pot of boiling water. Drain the boiling water and quickly shift the greens to a large bowl of ice water. Let the greens cool off, then strain, dry, and put aside. Melt butter and oil together in a wide saucepan over medium-high flame. Add the garlic and onions, then simmer for around 4-6 minutes, until lightly browned. Add the collard greens and the red and black pepper, then cook on high heat for 5-8 minutes, stirring continuously. Turn off the heat; if required, add vinegar, and stir

## 204 Honey Garlic Chicken

Preparation time: 1o minutes

Cooking Time: 60 minutes

Servings: 4

Difficulty Level: Easy

## Nutritional Information:

Calories: 279 kcal, protein: 13 g, carbohydrates: 36 g, Fat: 10 g, Cholesterol: 4o mg, Fiber: 0 g, Sodium: 40 mg, Potassium: 144 mg, Phosphorus: 99 mg, Calcium: 11 mg

## Ingredients:

- 1/2 cup of honey
- 4-pound of roasting chicken
- 1 teaspoon of garlic powder
- 1/2 teaspoon of black pepper
- 1 tablespoon of olive oil

## Instructions:

Preheat the oven to 350-degree F. Spray olive oil on a baking pan. Place chicken in the pan. Coat chicken with seasonings and honey. Bake until both sides are brown for 1 hour. During cooking, turn once.

## 205- Rosemary Chicken

Preparation time: 5 minutes

Cooking Time: 40 minutes

Servings: 4

Difficulty Level: Easy

## Nutritional Information:

Calories: 539 kcal, protein: 36.5 g, carbohydrates: 20 g, Fat: 32 g, Cholesterol: 117 mg, Fiber: 0.4 g, Sodium: 136 mg, Potassium: 412 mg, Phosphorus: 254 mg, Calcium: 49 mg

## Ingredients:

- 1/4 cup of oil such as canola or sunflower
- 1/3 cup of brown sugar
- 1 teaspoon of Worcestershire sauce
- 1 broiler-fryer chicken: split in half.
- 2 teaspoons of crushed, dried rosemary.
- 1/4 cup of lime juice
- 1/2 cup of dry, white wine

## Instructions:

To make a marinade, combine all the ingredients in a shallow dish, except chicken. Then add chicken and fold it thoroughly with marinade. Cover for at least 4 hours and refrigerate. Take out chicken, and for basting, reserve marinade. Place the chicken on the rack skin side in a broiling pan about 7 to 9 inches from the heating source, cook for 20 minutes and baste the chicken with marinade. Rotate chicken, apply marinade and broil generously for 15 minutes until soft.

## 206- Pasta with Cheesy Meat Sauce

Preparation time: 5 minutes

Cooking Time: 20 minutes

Servings: 6

Difficulty Level: Medium

## Nutritional Information:

Calories: 502 kcal, protein: 23 g, carbohydrates: 35 g, Fat: 30 g, Cholesterol: 99 mg, Fiber: 1.7 g, Sodium: 401 mg, Potassium: 549 mg, Phosphorus: 278 mg, Calcium: 107 mg

## Ingredients:

- 2 tablespoons of low-sodium Worcestershire sauce,
- ½ box of large-shaped pasta
- ½ cup of onions, diced.
- 1 pound of ground beef
- 1½ cups of beef stock, no sodium.
- 1 tablespoon of onion flakes
- ½ teaspoon of ground black pepper
- 1 tablespoon of tomato sauce, no salt.
- ¾ cup shredded Monterey or pepper jack cheese.
- 1 tablespoon of beef base, no salt.
- 8 ounces of cream cheese, softened.
- ½ teaspoon of Italian seasoning

## Instructions:

As per the instructions on the package, boil pasta noodles. Cook the onion flakes, ground beef, and onions in a large skillet until the meat is browned. Add tomato sauce, stock, and bouillon. Boil it, occasionally stir. Add cooked spaghetti, shredded cheese, cream cheese, and seasonings (Worcestershire sauce, black pepper, and Italian seasoning), and mix pasta until the cheese is melted.

## 207- Grilled Lemon Chicken Kebabs

Preparation time: 5 minutes

Cooking Time: 20 minutes

Servings: 2-3

Difficulty Level: Easy

## Nutritional Information:

Calories: 362 kcal, protein: 27 g, carbohydrates: 6 g, Fat: 0 g, Cholesterol: 5 mg, Fiber: 25 g, Sodium: 119 mg, Potassium: 404 mg, Phosphorus: 238 mg, Calcium: 30 mg

## Ingredients:

- 1 teaspoon of white vinegar
- 4 pieces of skinless, boneless chicken thighs
- 3 tablespoons of olive oil
- 2 lemons
- 1 clove of garlic crushed and peeled.
- 2 bay leaves (torn in half).
- 1 tablespoon of chopped fresh herbs (sage, thyme, etc.)

## Instructions:

Each thigh is sliced into chunks and placed in a bowl. Extract juice from lemons and grate only one tsp of lemon zest. Add oil, herbs, vinegar, lemon juice/ zest, garlic, and chicken to the cooking pan. For 3 hours, or overnight, marinate and cover it. Slice 4 thick slices of the other lemons, then slash each slice into 4 parts. The chicken pieces and the lemon slices are alternatively positioned on a wooden skewer, packed as close as possible, and the finish ends with a piece of lemon. For each skewer, repeat. Grill both sides in the oven or barbecue until cooked for 10 minutes.

## 208- Zesty Orange Tilapia

Preparation time: 10 minutes

Cooking Time: 20 minutes

Servings: 4

Difficulty Level: Easy

## Nutritional Information:

Calories: 133 kcal, protein: 24 g, carbohydrates: 6 g, Fat: 2 g, Cholesterol: 57 mg, Fiber: 1.7 g, Sodium: 97 mg, Potassium: 543 mg, Phosphorus: 214 mg, Calcium: 42 mg

## Ingredients:

- 4 teaspoons of orange juice
- 16 ounces of tilapia
- ¾ cup of celery, julienned
- 1 cup of carrots, julienned
- 2 teaspoons of grated orange peel (zest)
- 1 teaspoon of ground black pepper
- ½ cup of green onions, sliced.

## Instructions:

Preheat the oven to 450° F. Mix the celery, carrot, orange zest, and green onions in a shallow dish. Split 4 equal parts of the tilapia. Cut 4 wide foil squares and coat the foil with a non-adhesive spray.

Place 1/4 of the vegetables slightly on each foil section and cover with the fish. Sprinkle the surface of each one with 1 teaspoon of orange juice. Use ground black pepper for seasoning.

Make a pouch or envelope by wrapping foil, crimping the corners, and putting them on a baking sheet. Then bake for 12 minutes (if the fish is dense, 3-5 minutes longer). Take out pouches from the oven and place them directly on the dishes; when opening, be cautious because of the steam.

## 209- Simple Salmon Steaks

Preparation time: 5 minutes

Cooking Time: 20 minutes

Servings: 4

Difficulty Level: Easy

## Nutritional Information:

Calories: 392 kcal, protein: 34 g, carbohydrates: 3 g, Fat: 25.1 g, Cholesterol: 109.5 mg, Fiber: 0.3 g, Sodium: 150 mg, Potassium: 757 mg, Phosphorus: 504 mg, Calcium: 31 mg

## Ingredients:

- 4 6-ounce of salmon steaks
- 3 tablespoons of butter
- 1/2 teaspoon of lemon pepper
- 1 1/2 teaspoons of lemon juice
- 1/2 teaspoon of onion powder
- 1 teaspoon of dried tarragon crumbled.
- 1/2 teaspoon of garlic powder
- 2 lemon slices, halved.
- 1 teaspoon of paprika
- 4 thin onion slices
- 4 lemon wedges

## Instructions:

Brush melted butter on an 8×8" baking dish and place salmon on it. Sprinkle garlic powder, onion powder, lemon extract, and lemon pepper. Over salmon steaks, place a lemon piece and onion slices. Drizzle paprika and tarragon on it. Wrap it with a covering sheet and cook in the microwave on high settings for 6 minutes or until done. With lemon wedges, serve it.

## 210- Texas Hash

Preparation time: 5 minutes

Cooking Time: 1 hour 10 minutes

Servings: 8

Difficulty Level: Medium

## Nutritional Information:

Calories: 207 kcal, protein: 17 g, carbohydrates: 15 g, Fat: 2 g, Cholesterol: 5 mg, Fiber: 9 g, Sodium: 134 mg, Potassium: 427 mg, Phosphorus: 117 mg, Calcium: 133 mg

## Ingredients:

- 2 tablespoons of chili powder
- 1 (14.5 ounces) can of tomatoes: no salt (do not drain)
- 1 chopped onion.
- 1 1/2 pounds (24 ounces) of ground turkey
- 1/2 cup of rice
- 1 chopped green bell pepper.

## Instructions:

Preheat the oven to 350°F. Cook green peppers, onion, and turkey in a pan. Add the onion, tomatoes, rice, and chili powder when the turkey is cooked and the vegetables are soft (about 10-15 minutes). Place the mixture in a medium saucepan and cover it with foil. Bake for 40 minutes in the oven or 60 minutes if brown rice is used.

## 211- Rice with Chili Con Carne

Preparation time: 5 minutes

Cooking Time: 1 hour 30 minutes

Servings: 8

Difficulty Level: Easy

## Nutritional Information:

Calories: 190 kcal, protein: 20 g, carbohydrates: 5 g, Fat: 10 g, Cholesterol: 57 mg, Fiber: 1.25 g, Sodium: 116 mg, Potassium: 450 mg, Phosphorus: 180 mg, Calcium: 38 mg

## Ingredients:

- 3 cups of water
- 1-pound lean of ground beef
- 1 cup of chopped green pepper.
- 2 teaspoons of garlic powder
- 1 can (6 oz) tomato paste: no-salt
- 3-1/2 cups of cooked rice.
- 1 teaspoon of paprika

- 1 cup of chopped onion.
- 1/2 cup of cooked pinto beans (without salt)
- 1 teaspoon of ground cumin

## Instructions:

In a wide pan, cook the ground beef until it turns brown; remove extra oil. Add the green pepper and onion and cook; add all left ingredients and cook for 1-1/2 hours. Serve with hot rice.

## 212- Pizza

Preparation time: 5 minutes

Cooking Time: 35 minutes

Servings: 6

Difficulty Level: Easy

## Nutritional Information:

Calories: 402 kcal, protein: 22 g, carbohydrates: 38 g, Fat: 18 g, Cholesterol: 50 mg, Fiber: 2.8 g, Sodium: 150 mg, Potassium: 352 mg, Phosphorus: 230 mg, Calcium: 236 mg

## Ingredients:

**For Dough**

- 2 cups of flour
- 1 tbsp of oil
- 1 cup of water (water)
- 1 tbsp sugar
- 1/2 package of dry yeast

**Sauce**

- 6 oz mozzarella cheese, shredded.
- 1/4 cup chopped green pepper.
- 1/2 cup water
- 1 tablespoon oil
- 1/2 lb. ground beef cooked, well-drained.
- 1/4 teaspoon of garlic powder
- 1/2 teaspoon of oregano
- 3 oz tomato paste: no-salt

- 1/4 cup of chopped onion.
- 1 tablespoon of sugar

## Instructions:

In warm water, add yeast. To make a smooth dough, mix flour,1 tablespoon of sugar, and 1 tablespoon of oil. Knead it accordingly. Put a greased bowl, cover it, and leave it to set in a warm area. In a shallow saucepan, add the garlic powder, 1/2 cup water, tomato paste, oregano, 1 tablespoon oil, and 1 tablespoon sugar. Simmer for 5 mins.

Grease a baking sheet that is 17 x 14-inch. Spread dough over sheet towards edges. Use sauce to coat the dough. Place the green pepper, onion, cheese, and beef on top. For 20 to 30 minutes, bake at 400 ° F until the cheese and dough are golden browns. Slice into 12 pieces.

## 213- Vegetable Curry

Preparation time: 30 minutes

Cooking Time: 30 minutes

Servings: 5

Difficulty Level: Easy

## Nutritional Information:

Calories: 318 kcal, protein: 6 g, carbohydrates: 30 g, Fat: 20 g, Cholesterol: 0 mg, Fiber: 4 g, Sodium: 33 mg, Potassium: 477 mg, Phosphorus: 175 mg, Calcium: 58 mg

## Ingredients:

- 2 cups of basmati rice
- 1 teaspoon of cumin seeds, whole
- ¼ teaspoon of black peppercorns, whole
- 1 teaspoon of mustard seeds, whole
- 1 teaspoon of coriander seeds, whole
- 1 teaspoon of fennel seeds, whole
- 1 (2-inch) piece of ginger grated finely.
- 1 tablespoon of coconut oil
- ½ teaspoon of hot chili flakes

- 1 teaspoon of turmeric
- 1 can of coconut milk
- 1 medium (70g) quartered onion.
- 1 cup of green peas, frozen
- 1½ cups of cauliflower: bite-sized florets.
- 1 medium diced (61g) carrot.

## Instructions:

In an iron skillet, fry dry spices for 2 minutes over low to medium heat. Boil rice according to the package instructions. Sauté spices in coconut oil until slightly browned and popping, for around 2-3 minutes over low to medium heat. Then add the turmeric, hot chili flakes, and ginger. Cook for 6 minutes over low to medium heat until aromatic. Take off the heat, combine the onion and cooked spices in a blender, and make a paste. Heat the coconut milk in a separate pan until it bubbles and add the seasoning paste; whisk thoroughly. Add prepared vegetables and cook for around 10 minutes until they are soft. Serve over rice.

## 214 Brewery Burger

Preparation time: 5 minutes

Cooking Time: 20-30 minutes

Servings: 4

Difficulty Level: Easy

## Nutritional Information:

Calories: 242 kcal, protein: 22 g, carbohydrates: 7 g, Fat: 14 g, Cholesterol: 116 mg, Fiber: 0.2 g, Sodium: 92 mg, Potassium: 328 mg, Phosphorus: 188 mg, Calcium: 31 mg

## Ingredients:

- 5 soda crackers: salt-free
- 3 tablespoons of rice milk
- 1 pound of ground beef, 85% lean
- 1 large egg

- 1 teaspoon of herb seasoning blend: salt-free

## Instructions:

Break soda crackers into fine pieces and then mix them in a cup with the milk. Let the crackers stay in it until they are soft. Beat and whisk an egg with a cracker mixture, add ground beef and herbs, and mix thoroughly. Make four ground beef patties of the same size. Grill until cooked over medium heat; the internal temperature should be at least 160° F. Serve on a baguette with vegetables and favorite toppings.

## 215- Persian Chicken

Preparation time:  1 hour 30 minutes

Cooking Time: 20 minutes

Servings: 5

Difficulty Level: Easy

## Nutritional Information:

Calories: 330 kcal, protein: 22 g, carbohydrates: 3 g, Fat: 23 g, Cholesterol: 107 mg, Fiber: 1 g, Sodium: 102 mg, Potassium: 333 mg, Phosphorus: 214 mg, Calcium: 25 mg

## Ingredients:

- 2 tbsp of dried oregano
- 10 skinless, boneless chicken thighs
- 1 onion: large chopped.
- 2 tsp of sweet paprika
- 1 cup of olive oil
- ½ cup of fresh lemon juice
- 2 tsp of minced garlic

## Instructions:

Add lemon juice, onion, paprika, garlic, and oregano to the jar of a food processor and blend it. Then add the oil slowly to the jar while it's blending. Put the chicken in a wide plastic bag that can be resealed, and pour the marinade.

Seal it firmly by pressing out air. Refrigerate over for 1 hour and make sure chicken is well marinated. Take out the chicken and discard the excess marinade. For approximately 10 minutes, barbeque it over direct medium fire, rotating once. Make sure it's fully cooked inside. Serve with rice and vegetable salad.

## 216- Turkey Sloppy Joes

Preparation time: 10 minutes

Cooking Time: 20 minutes

Servings: 6

Difficulty Level: Easy

## Nutritional Information:

Calories: 290 kcal, protein: 24 g, carbohydrates: 28 g, Fat: 9 g, Cholesterol: 58 mg, Fiber: 1.8 g, Sodium: 288 mg, Potassium: 513 mg, Phosphorus: 237 mg, Calcium: 86 mg

## Ingredients:

- 6 hamburger buns
- 1/2 cup of red onion
- 1-1/2 pounds of ground turkey, 7% fat
- 1/2 cup of green bell pepper
- 2 tablespoons of brown sugar
- 1 tablespoon of Chicken Grilling Blend seasoning
- 1 cup of tomato sauce: low-sodium
- 1 tablespoon of Worcestershire sauce

## Instructions:

Chop the bell pepper and onion. Add turkey onion and bell peppering wide skillet and cook over medium-high heat. Mix cinnamon, spice, tomato sauce, and Worcestershire sauce in a small bowl. Then mix this blend with turkey. Lower the flame and cook for 10 minutes. Serve with hamburger buns.

# 217- Fast Fajitas

Preparation time: 5 minutes

Cooking Time: 30 minutes

Servings: 4

Difficulty Level: Easy

## Nutritional Information:

Calories: 320 kcal, protein: 29 g, carbohydrates: 34 g, Fat: 5 g, Cholesterol: 53 mg, Fiber: 8 g, Sodium: 142 mg, Potassium: 445 mg, Phosphorus: 332 mg, Calcium: 23 mg

## Ingredients:

- Eight corn tortillas
- 1 tablespoon of olive oil
- cayenne pepper
- 1 lemon juice and zest of lemon or orange
- 1 pound of meat: bite-size pieces (shrimp, Tofu)
- 1 onion, sliced.
- 1 teaspoon of cumin
- 2 sliced bell peppers.
- Cilantro to taste
- sour cream to taste.

## Instructions:

To make the marinade, combine citrus juice, zest, oil, cayenne pepper, and cumin in a shallow bowl. Put vegetables, marinade, and meat in a small bowl, cover it and marinate it overnight. Cook marinated vegetables and meat for 15-20 minutes in a wide skillet over medium heat until the onions become soft and light brown and the meat becomes tender. Serve with tortillas and cover with cilantro and sour cream.

# 218- Jambalaya

Preparation time: 5 minutes

Cooking Time: 1 hour 15 minutes

Servings: 12

Difficulty Level: Easy

## Nutritional Information:

Calories: 294 kcal, protein: 20 g, carbohydrates: 31 g, Fat: 10 g, Cholesterol: 137 mg, Fiber: 0.8 g, Sodium: 186 mg, Potassium: 300 mg, Phosphorus: 197 mg, Calcium: 65 mg

## Ingredients:

- 8 ounces tomato sauce: low-sodium(canned)
- 2 cups of onion
- 1/2 teaspoon of black pepper
- 1 cup of bell pepper
- 2 cups of beef broth: low-sodium
- 2 garlic cloves
- 1/2 cup of margarine
- 2 pounds of raw shrimp
- 2 cups of white rice, uncooked.

## Instructions:

Preheat the oven to 350° F. Chop the garlic, onion, and bell pepper. Scrape shrimp. Mix all ingredients in a large bowl except margarine. Pour it into a 9-inch x 13-inch baking dish and evenly spread it. Sprinkle margarine and cover it and bake for 1 hr. and 15 minutes. Serve it hot.

# 219- Halibut with Lemon Caper Sauce

Preparation time: 5 minutes

Cooking Time: 20 minutes

Servings: 6

Difficulty Level: Easy

## Nutritional Information:

Calories: 340 kcal, protein: 26 g, carbohydrates: 34 g, Fat: 9 g, Cholesterol: 46 mg, Fiber: 0.6 g, Sodium: 118 mg, Potassium: 573 mg, Phosphorus: 307 mg, Calcium: 79 mg

## Ingredients:

- 4 cups of cooked white rice.
- 3 tablespoons of lemon juice
- 10 ounces of halibut steaks
- 1 tablespoon of olive oil
- 1 cup of low-sodium chicken broth.
- 3 tablespoons of unsalted butter
- 1/3 cup of white vinegar
- 3 teaspoons of white flour: all-purpose
- 1/4 teaspoon of white pepper
- 1-1/2 teaspoons of capers

## Instructions:

In a sealable bag, add halibut,1 tablespoon olive oil, and lemon juice; marinate for five minutes. Use cooking spray to grease a non-stick skillet and heat it. Cook halibut in it for three minutes. Flip it and cook for two more minutes, then take it out.

Melt butter over low heat in the pan for sauce making, add flour and chicken broth and whisk for 1 minute. Add lemon juice, pepper, and capers. Stir for 3 to 5 minutes until sauce gets thick. To reheat, put the halibut in a skillet with the sauce. Divide the fish into four pieces and serve with 1/4-cup sauce spooned over the fish and cooked rice.

## 220- Pesto Chicken

Preparation time: 10 minutes

Cooking Time: 6-8 hours

Servings: 8

Difficulty Level: Easy

## Nutritional Information:

Calories: 340 kcal, protein: 25 g, carbohydrates: 33 g, Fat: 12 g, Cholesterol: 59 mg, Fiber: 2.9 g, Sodium: 322 mg, Potassium: 450 mg, Phosphorus: 257 mg, Calcium: 40 mg

## Ingredients:

- ½ cup of low-sodium chicken (or veggie) broth
- 6-ounce jar of pesto
- 3 chicken breast fillets

## Instructions:

Put chicken breasts in the slow cooker and add pesto over it. Then pour 1/2 cup of chicken broth into it. Cook for 6-8 hours on LOW. Serve with pasta.

## 221- Balsamic Chicken Thighs

Preparation time: 5 minutes

Cooking Time: 6-8 hours

Servings: 8

Difficulty Level: Easy

## Nutritional Information:

Calories: 211 kcal, protein: 30 g, carbohydrates: 7 g, Fat: 7 g, Cholesterol: 73 mg, Fiber: 0.5 g, Sodium: 88 mg, Potassium: 337 mg, Phosphorus: 230 mg, Calcium: 34 mg

## Ingredients:

- 1 teaspoon of garlic powder
- 8 chicken thighs
- ½ teaspoon of salt
- 1 teaspoon of dried basil
- 4 minced garlic cloves.
- ½ teaspoon of pepper
- 2 teaspoons of dried minced onion
- 1 Tablespoon of olive oil
- Fresh chopped parsley
- ½ cup of balsamic vinegar

## Instructions:

Mix garlic powder, dried basil, salt, pepper, and dried minced onions in a small bowl and coat the chicken. Add garlic and olive oil to the slow cooker. Then add chicken and pour vinegar over it. Cook for 6-8 hours on LOW. Garnish fresh parsley and serve with noodles.

## 222- Spicy Coconut Curry Chicken

Preparation time: 10 minutes

Cooking Time: 7-9 hours 30 minutes

Servings: 2-3

Difficulty Level: Easy

### Nutritional Information:

Calories: 348 kcal, protein: 40 g, carbohydrates: 19 g, Fat: 12 g, Cholesterol: 70 mg, Fiber: 3 g, Sodium: 239 mg, Potassium: 557 mg, Phosphorus: 332.7 mg, Calcium: 168 mg

### Ingredients:

- ¼ cup green onions: chopped.
- 2 chicken breasts: boneless (fresh or frozen)
- 2 Tablespoons of minced garlic
- 1 (4 ounces) can of green chili peppers: dice.
- 1 Tablespoon of chili powder
- 1 ½ Tablespoon of curry powder
- ½ teaspoon of cinnamon
- 1 teaspoon of cumin
- 1 ½ cup of water
- 1 Tablespoon of lime juice
- 1 (7 ounces) can of coconut milk
- Chopped cilantro for garnish.
- 1 cup of dry white rice

### Instruction:

Add all ingredients to the slow cooker except rice and coconut milk. Cover it and cook for 7-9 hours on LOW. Shred the chicken with a fork once cooked and whisk in dry rice and coconut milk. Switch the slow cooker to HIGH. Cook for 30 minutes until the liquid is absorbed and the rice is cooked. Garnish with cilantro and serve hot.

## 223- Chicken Curry

Preparation time: 5 minutes

Cooking Time: 30 minutes

Servings: 6

Difficulty Level: Easy

### Nutritional Information:

Calories: 323 kcal, protein: 21 g, carbohydrates: 5 g, Fat: 24 g, Cholesterol: 5 mg, Fiber: 3 g, Sodium: 93 mg, Potassium: 317 mg, Phosphorus: 214 mg, Calcium: 25 mg

### Ingredients:

- 6 skinless, boneless chicken thighs
- 3 tablespoons of olive oil, divided.
- 2 teaspoons of minced garlic
- 1 small, sweet onion
- 1 tablespoon of Hot Curry Powder
- 2 tablespoons of chopped fresh cilantro.
- 1 teaspoon of grated fresh ginger
- ¼ cup of coconut milk
- ¾ cup of water

### Instructions:

In a large skillet over medium-high heat, heat 2 tablespoons of the oil. Add the chicken and cook for about 10 minutes or until the thighs are browned. With tongs, remove the chicken to a plate and set it aside. Add the remaining 1 tablespoon of oil to the skillet and sauté the onion, garlic, and ginger for about 3 minutes or until they are softened. Add coconut milk curry powder and water. Put the chicken in a pan and boil the liquid. Lower the heat, cover the pan, and simmer for about 25 minutes or until the chicken is tender and the sauce is thick. Serve topped with cilantro.

## 224- Garlic Green Beans

Preparation time: 5 minutes

Cooking Time: 40 minutes

Servings: 6

Difficulty Level: Easy

### Nutritional Information:

Calories: 102 kcal, protein: 2 g, carbohydrates: 6 g, Fat: 4 g, Cholesterol: 10 mg, Fiber: 1.7 g, Sodium: 2 mg, Potassium: 107 mg, Phosphorus: 22 mg, Calcium: 48 mg

### Ingredients:

- 1 cup of boiling water
- 2 lbs. of green beans, trimmed.
- 1/4 cup of butter or margarine
- 1/2 tsp. of salt
- Four garlic cloves pressed.
- 1/4 cup of fresh parsley: chopped.
- 1/4 tsp. of lemon pepper

### Instructions:

Put the salt, water, and green bean in a Dutch oven, cover and cook for 30 minutes over medium heat and drain it. In a Dutch oven, melt the butter, add the lemon pepper and garlic, and sauté the mixture over medium heat for 1 to 2 minutes. Add the green beans and stir-fry for 5 minutes. Garnish parsley.

## 225- Chili Rice with Beef

Preparation time: 5 minutes

Cooking Time: 30 minutes

Servings: 4

Difficulty Level: Easy

### Nutritional Information:

Calories: 386 kcal, protein: 27 g, carbohydrates: 38 g, Fat: 14 g, Cholesterol: 75 mg, Fiber: 2.3 g, Sodium: 300 mg, Potassium: 552 mg, Phosphorus: 278 mg, Calcium: 53 mg

### Ingredients:

- 1-pound of lean ground beef
- Two tablespoons of vegetable oil
- 1 cup of onion, chopped.
- 1 ½ teaspoon of chili con carne seasoning powder
- Two cups of rice, cooked.
- ½ teaspoon of sage
- ⅛ teaspoon of black pepper

### Instructions:

Warm oil; add onion and beef. Cook until browned and keep stirring. Add seasonings and rice. Mix them. Take it off from the heat. Cover them and make them stand for 10-14 mins.

## 226- Baked Tuna

Preparation time: 10 minutes

Cooking Time: 20 minutes

Servings: 4

Difficulty Level: Easy

### Nutritional Information:

Calories: 277 kcal, protein: 40 g, carbohydrates: 1 g, Fat: 12 g, Cholesterol: 65 mg, Fiber: 1 g, Sodium: 357 mg, Potassium: 434 mg, Phosphorus: 183 mg, Calcium: 16 mg

### Ingredients:

- 2/3 cup of chopped onion.
- 14 oz. of Canned Tuna in water, no salt.
- 1/4 cup of canned pimento
- 1/4 cup of a green pepper diced.

- 2 Tablespoons of Parmesan cheese: grated.
- 1/2 cup of mayonnaise
- non-stick cooking spray
- 1/4 cup of plain breadcrumbs

## Instructions:

Set oven to 350°F. Spray a baking dish with non-stick cooking spray. Combine the onion, Tuna, pepper, mayonnaise, and pimento e in a wide bowl. Put the mixture of Tuna in a baking dish. Sprinkle with Parmesan cheese and breadcrumbs. Bake for 20 minutes (or until heated thoroughly), and the top is light brown.

## 227- Fried White Pomfret

Preparation time: 1 hour 5 minutes

Cooking Time: 20 minutes

Servings: 3-4

Difficulty Level: Easy

## Nutritional Information:

Calories: 87 kcal, protein: 24 g, carbohydrates: 1.8 g, Fat: 15 g, Cholesterol: 46 mg, Fiber: 2.9 g, Sodium: 145 mg, Potassium: 65.5 mg, Phosphorus: 12 mg, Calcium: 200 mg

## Ingredients:

- 1 tsp of turmeric powder
- 600–800g white pomfret, washed and gutted
- 2 tsp of salt
- 20g ginger, thinly sliced.
- 1 medium onion, chopped.
- Two cloves of garlic, minced.
- 1 tsp of chili powder
- 2 tbsp of cumin
- 1 tsp of coriander seed
- 150ml of water
- Two small tomatoes, chopped.
- 60ml of vegetable oil

- ¾ tsp of sugar (optional)
- Salt/pepper season to taste.
- 30ml of lemon juice

## Instructions:

Marinate the fish for 1 hour with salt and turmeric powder. Add some oil and sauté the ginger, onion, garlic, cumin, coriander seeds, tomatoes, and chili powder in a hot pan. Deglaze the pan with water and lemon juice until the onion is softened and spices are well mixed. Put in the sugar and season the sauce. Pan-fry fish with oil until brown and cooked thoroughly. Serve the fish warm and lay the sauce on top of it.

## 228- Steamed Silver Pomfret Teochew Style

Preparation time: 2 hours

Cooking Time: 15 minutes

Servings: 4

Difficulty Level: Easy

## Nutritional Information:

Calories: 483 kcal, protein: 76 g, carbohydrates: 23 g, Fat: 10g, Cholesterol: 5 mg, Fiber: 4 g, Sodium: 31 mg, Potassium: 139 mg, Phosphorus: 12 mg, Calcium: 7 mg

## Ingredients:

- 1/4 cup of carrot, shredded.
- 10g ginger, thinly sliced.
- One small-sized tomato: wedged.
- A few sprigs of coriander leaves
- 1/2 small-sized red chili: thinly sliced.
- 1/4 cup of scallion, chopped.
- 450–600g of pomfret, cleaned and gutted
- Salt/pepper season to taste.
- 1 1/2 tbsps. Of soya sauce, light

## Instructions:

Rub salt and pepper on whole fish. Leave it to marinate for 2 hours in the refrigerator before steaming. Depending on the size, steam the fish for 12-14 minutes with all remaining ingredients. Serve it hot.

## 229- Grilled Mexican Snapper Fillet

Preparation time: 45 minutes

Cooking Time: 15 minutes

Servings: 4

Difficulty Level: Easy

## Nutritional Information:

Calories: 218 kcal, protein: 45 g, carbohydrates: 0 g, Fat: 2.9 g, Cholesterol: 80 mg, Fiber: 0 g, Sodium: 97 mg, Potassium: 887 mg, Phosphorus: 531 mg, Calcium: 28 mg

## Ingredients:

- 4 cups of Chinese parsley, fresh
- 100g of snapper fillets, three pieces
- 4 cups of white onion, chopped.
- 2 tbsp of sugar
- 1 tbsp of chopped green chili, seeds removed.
- 4 cups of lime juice
- One clove garlic
- Salt/pepper season to taste.
- 2 tbsp of canola oil

## Instructions:

Mix Chinese parsley, salt, sugar, onion, lime juice, chili, garlic, and oil until smooth in a blender or food processor. Pour the paste over the fish, and coat it on both sides. Marinate and keep for at least 45 minutes in the refrigerator. Pan-fry the fish on both sides for around 5 to 7 minutes or until the fish breaks easily with a fork. Garnish with wedges of lime and serve it.

## 230- Lamb Chops with Redcurrant and Mint Sauce

Preparation time: 5 minutes

Cooking Time: 50 minutes

Servings: 2

Difficulty Level: Easy

## Nutritional Information:

Calories: 436.2 kcal, protein: 48.6 g, carbohydrates: 2.3 g, Fat: 24.5 g, Cholesterol: 151.5 mg, Fiber: 0.8 g, Sodium: 177.1 mg, Potassium: 697.5 mg, Phosphorus: 456.9 mg, Calcium: 82.5 mg

## Ingredients:

- 1tbsp of Mint sauce
- 4tbsp of Redcurrant jelly
- 4tbsp of Water
- 4 Lean lamb chops (approx. 140g each): cut.
- 1tbsp of Lemon juice

## Instructions:

Mix the mint sauce, redcurrant jelly, water, and lemon juice in an ovenproof bowl. Trim the chops and place the sauce in the bowl; turn each chop to coat well. Bake uncovered at 180°F in a pre-heated oven for 35-40 minutes until the lamb is tender. Before serving. Add corn flour and a small amount of water to make the sauce thick. Serve with boiled potatoes and vegetables.

## 231- Plant-based Bean Bourguignon

Preparation time: 5 minutes

Cooking Time:50 minutes

Servings: 4

Difficulty Level: Medium

## Nutritional Information:

Calories: 214.7 kcal, protein: 8.6 g, carbohydrates: 42.3 g, Fat: 4.2 g, Cholesterol: 6 mg, Fiber: 8.8 g, Sodium: 201.2 mg, Potassium: 676.42 mg, Phosphorus: 73.39 mg, Calcium: 64 mg

## Ingredients:

- Three cups of Vegetable stock: no salt.
- 1 Tbsp of Garlic, fresh, minced.
- 4 Medium onions: diced.
- ¼ Cup of Cannellini Beans, drained
- 1 medium diced Carrot,
- One can (425g) of Black Beans: no salt, canned, drained.
- 1 Tbsp of Olive oil
- 20g Parsley: chopped.
- ½ tsp of Black pepper
- 1 tsp of smoked paprika
- Three sprigs of thyme, fresh
- 4 Tbsp of Flour, all-purpose

## Instructions:

Add oil and fry onions until lightly browned in a Dutch oven or a pot. Stir in the garlic and carrots, gently sauté the mushrooms, and put them aside. Add thyme, pepper, flour, and smoked paprika. Deglaze the pan with a splash of vegetable stock. Switch to medium-high heat, add the remaining vegetable stock, and mix until thickened. Take off from the heat. When cooking, scrub the bottom to remove all the pieces from the bottom of the pot. Then beans are added. Cook until carrots are tender for around 30 minutes. Hold the pot uncovered when simmering. Sprinkle parsley and serve it.

## 232- Lamb and Ginger Stir Fry

Preparation time: 5 minutes

Cooking Time: 20 minutes

Servings: 2

Difficulty Level: Easy

## Nutritional Information:

Calories: 336 kcal, protein: 24 g, carbohydrates: 13 g, Fat: 21 g, Cholesterol: 82 mg, Fiber: 3.1 g, Sodium: 532 mg, Potassium: 550 mg, Phosphorus: 272 mg, Calcium: 26 mg

## Ingredients:

- 1tbsp of cooked peas
- 1tsp of Ginger root, chopped.
- 225g of Minced lamb
- Pepper
- A little sunflower oil

## Instructions:

Fry the lamb for 3-4 minutes or until browned in the sunflower oil. Add the ginger and cook for a further 2-3 minutes. Add pepper and peas. Serve with noodles or rice.

## 233- Ham and beans

Preparation time: 25 minutes

Cooking Time: 50 minutes

Servings: 6

Difficulty Level: Medium

## Nutritional Information:

Calories: 293 kcal, protein: 12 g, carbohydrates: 42 g, Fat: 9 g, Cholesterol: 9 mg, Fiber: 3 g, Sodium: 305 mg, Potassium: 477 mg, Phosphorus: 182 mg, Calcium: 40 mg

## Ingredients:

- 3 Tbsp of oil
- 1/2 cup of low sodium ham
- 1.5 cups of onion, diced.
- 1 cup of baby lima beans, raw
- Four garlic cloves
- 1 cup of white or brown rice, raw

- 2 tbsp of cider vinegar
- 1/2 tsp of smoked paprika
- 1 tbsp of honey
- 1/4 tsp of salt
- 32 oz of chicken broth: low sodium
- 2 jalapeno peppers (opt)
- 1/2 tsp of ground pepper

## Instructions:

Add low sodium chicken broth and 2 cups of water to the pressure cooker with beans and rice. Cook as pressure cooker directions (45 minutes at pressure and then 20 minutes natural release for unsoaked beans)

Chop and sauté the onion and garlic in oil while the beans are boiling. Add the honey, vinegar, salt, paprika, jalapenos, and pepper to a small bowl to make a seasoning blend. Add the garlic, onion, the seasoning mix, and ham into the rice and beans once they are done. Mix to combine thoroughly. Serve with chives.

## 234- Pesto Pronto

Preparation time: 5 minutes

Cooking Time: 20 minutes

Servings: 6

Difficulty Level: Easy

## Nutritional Information:

Calories: 472 kcal, protein: 14 g, carbohydrates: 64 g, Fat: 18 g, Cholesterol: 8 mg, Fiber: 5 g, Sodium: 341 mg, Potassium: 516 mg, Phosphorus: 87 mg, Calcium: 110 mg

## Ingredients:

- Two medium Zucchini: sliced in half.
- 16 oz of White Pasta
- One medium Yellow Squash is sliced in half.
- 1/2 cup of Mushrooms: sliced thick.

- 1 Large Red Bell Pepper, diced inch squares
- 2 tbsp of Olive Oil
- 1/4 cup of Feta Cheese
- 2/3 cup of Pesto Sauce
- 2 cloves Garlic

## Instructions:

Preheat the oven to 425 degrees F. Add the squash, zucchini, onion, mushrooms, bell, and pepper on a baking sheet of 18 to 13 inches. Drizzle the vegetables with olive oil and flip to cover them uniformly. Roast the vegetables in a pre-heated oven until soft. When roasting vegetables, cook pasta according to the packet and rinse. Into a large bowl, add drained spaghetti. Add the roasted vegetables and pesto to layer uniformly, then toss. Serve it hot.

## 235- Thai Shrimp Kebabs

Preparation time: 1 hour 10 minutes

Cooking Time: 25 minutes

Servings: 8

Difficulty Level: Easy

## Nutritional Information:

Calories: 157 kcal, protein: 18 g, carbohydrates: 8 g, Fat: 5 g, Cholesterol: 128 mg, Fiber: 1 g, Sodium: 150 mg, Potassium: 374 mg, Phosphorus: 206 mg, Calcium: 105 mg

## Ingredients:

- Two cups of cauliflower cut into florets.
- One cup of red pepper, cubed.
- Two small onions, quartered.
- ½ cup of fresh lime juice
- 1 tbsp of red or green Thai curry paste
- ½ cup of white wine
- ⅓ cup of fresh basil
- ½ cup of vegetable oil
- Eight skewers

- 1 ½ lb. of shelled raw shrimp.

## Instructions:

Slice the red peppers, cauliflower, and onions. Place the cauliflower for 2 minutes in boiling water, drain and set aside. Whisk together the lime juice, vinegar, oil, spices, and curry paste in a bowl. Mix shrimp and all the vegetables with the mixture. Refrigerate for at least 1 hour. Place the shrimp and vegetables on skewers. Barbecue it on medium heat for 15-18 minutes, rotating once and serving it once done.

## 236- Frittatas

Preparation time: 5 minutes

Cooking Time: 30 minutes

Servings: 4

Difficulty Level: Medium

## Nutritional Information:

Calories: 87 kcal, protein: 8 g, carbohydrates: 7 g, Fat: 3 g, Cholesterol: 106 mg, Fiber: 2.3 g, Sodium: 184 mg, Potassium: 360 mg, Phosphorus: 96 mg, Calcium: 38 mg

## Ingredients:

- 2-3 tbsp of fresh basil, diced.
- ⅓ cup of red bell pepper, diced.
- ¼ cup of shredded cheese
- and ⅓ cup of Zucchini, diced.
- ¼ tsp of pepper
- ⅓ cup of broccoli, chopped.
- 10-12 eggs
- ½ tsp of seasoning of choice (optional): salt-free

## Instructions:

Preheat the oven to 375 degrees F. Spray oil on a 12-cup muffin pan. Combine Zucchini, red bell pepper, basil, and broccoli in a medium dish. Whisk together the pepper, eggs, cheese, and salt-free seasoning in a wide bowl. Combine the egg mixture with a veggie mixture and whisk. Fill muffin cups with egg mixture (about 1/4 to 1/3 cup each) using a measuring cup. For 18 to 20 minutes, bake the egg muffins until the eggs are cooked in the center. Muffins can be stored for up to 3 to 4 days in an airtight jar in the fridge.

## 237- Jalapeno Pepper Chicken

Preparation time: 10 minutes

Cooking Time: 40 minutes

Servings: 4-5

Difficulty Level: Easy

## Nutritional Information:

Calories: 279 kcal, protein: 13 g, carbohydrates: 36 g, Fat: 10 g, Cholesterol: 5 mg, Fiber: 0 g, Sodium: 40 mg, Potassium: 144 mg, Phosphorus: 99 mg, Calcium: 80 mg

## Ingredients:

- 2 teaspoons of finely chopped, fresh jalapeño peppers and seeded.
- 2-3 pounds of chicken, cut up (skin and fat removed)
- 3 tablespoons of vegetable oil
- 1 onion sliced into rings.
- ½ teaspoon of ground nutmeg
- 1 ½ cups of chicken bouillon; low-sodium
- ¼ teaspoon of black pepper

## Instructions:

Heat oil, cook chicken until brown, and put aside. Keep it warm. In the same oil, add onions and sauté. Add the bouillon and boil it, occasionally stirring. Return the chicken to the pan; add black pepper and nutmeg. Cover and cook until the chicken is tender, or for 35 minutes. Add the jalapeño peppers, cook for a minute, and serve warm.

## 238- Salisbury Steak

Preparation time: 5 minutes

Cooking Time: 30 minutes

Servings: 4

Difficulty Level: Medium

### Nutritional Information:

Calories: 94 kcal, protein: 4.4 g, carbohydrates: 4.3 g, Fat: 6.6 g, Cholesterol: 21 mg, Fiber: 0.6 g, Sodium: 321 mg, Potassium: 91 mg, Phosphorus: 144 mg, Calcium: 30 mg

### Ingredients:

- 1 small onion, chopped.
- 1-pound lean ground chicken, beef, or turkey chopped steak.
- 1 teaspoon of black pepper
- 1 tablespoon of corn starch
- ½ cup of chopped green pepper.
- 1 egg
- ½ cup of water
- 1 tablespoon of vegetable oil

### Instructions:

Blend meat, green pepper, onion, egg, and black pepper in a bowl. Shape it into patties. In a pan, heat oil, add patties, and cook each side. Pour half of the water and allow it for 15 minutes to boil. Remove the patties. Add the remaining water and corn starch to the meat drippings. Simmer to thicken the sauce while stirring. Over steak, pour gravy, and serve hot.

## 239- Fried Gnocchi with Broccoli and Peas

Preparation time: 10 minutes

Cooking Time: 20 minutes

Servings: 4

Difficulty Level: Easy

### Nutritional Information:

Calories: 157 kcal, protein: 4 g, carbohydrates: 12 g, Fat: 11 g, Cholesterol: 5 mg, Fiber: 3 g, Sodium: 378 mg, Potassium: 325 mg, Phosphorus: 109.9 mg, Calcium: 42 mg

### Ingredients:

- 1 medium-small sliced yellow onion (about 1 cup)
- 1-pound of prepared gnocchi
- 4 tablespoons of olive oil: extra-virgin
- ½ cup of frozen peas
- 2 cups of chopped broccoli (frozen or fresh)
- The ¼-½ cup of water
- 2 cloves of diced garlic.
- ¼-½ teaspoons of red pepper flakes
- 2 tablespoons of lemon juice
- 2 tablespoons of Parmigiano-Reggiano: grated.
- 1 teaspoon of lemon zest,

### Instructions:

Boil water in a large saucepan. Add gnocchi and cook it until it floats. Drain it. Meanwhile, heat 2 tablespoons of oil in a large (preferably 12-inch) non-stick skillet over medium heat and cook the onion until it begins to brown. Add garlic and broccoli. Stir and sauté, then cover the mixture for approximately 5 minutes until the broccoli is done. Add the pepper flakes and frozen peas and cook for 2-3 minutes. Then add lemon zest and juice and set this combination aside. Add 2 tablespoons of oil and gnocchi to the skillet. Fry Gnocchi for around 5 -10 minutes over medium-high flame until it browns on both sides. Add pea mixture, onion, broccoli, and Parmigiano, and mix them. Cover the gnocchi with 1/4 to 1/2 cup water (about 4 tablespoons) for moistening. Serve it.

# 240- Three Cheese Veggie Lasagna

Preparation time: 10 minutes

Cooking Time: 1 hour 20 minutes

Servings: 8

Difficulty Level: Medium

## Nutritional Information:

Calories: 487 kcal, protein: 25 g, carbohydrates: 45 g, Fat: 23 g, Cholesterol: 100 mg, Fiber: 2.8 g, Sodium: 214 mg, Potassium: 492 mg, Phosphorus: 242 mg, Calcium: 110 mg

## Ingredients:

- 1 onion, diced.
- 2 teaspoons of olive oil
- 1 yellow squash, cubed.
- 5-ounce bag of kale-broccoli slaw (or shredded kale)
- 3 cups of milk: fat-free
- 3 cloves garlic, crushed.
- ½ cup of shredded Swiss cheese: low fat
- 1 15-ounce container of ricotta cheese: fat-free
- Ground green pepper as a garnish.
- Three tablespoons of parmesan cheese
- One package of no-boil lasagna; is divided into thirds.
- 3 tablespoons of all-purpose flour

## Instructions:

Set the oven to 375 degrees F. Use a non-stick cooking spray to coat a 9x13-inch baking dish (olive oil is best used as a cooking spray). Heat oil over medium to high heat in a wide non-stick skillet. Add squash and onion; cook until lightly browned, stirring regularly, for 8 minutes. Add kale and garlic; continuously stir until softened, for 3 minutes at least. Take it off from heat; allow it to cool for five minutes. Add Swiss, ricotta, and parmesan cheeses until well combined. Put aside. Mix the milk and flour in a medium saucepan until thick to make the sauce. Cook continually, whisking over medium heat until the sauce starts to bubble and thickens. It will require eight minutes. Layer the baking dish with ingredients: In the bottom of the bowl, place 1/3 of the noodles and then top with 1/2 of the veggie combination over the noodles; repeat with the rest. The leftover sauce will cover the last layer of 1/3 noodles and the top sheet. With foil, cover the lasagna loosely, and bake for 45 minutes. Remove the foil and cook until it bubbles; for 10 minutes. Let it stand before serving for 10 minutes.

# 241- Cream Cheese Chicken Chili

Preparation time: 10 minutes

Cooking Time: 8 hours

Servings: 8

Difficulty Level: Easy

## Nutritional Information:

Calories: 355 kcal, protein: 24 g, carbohydrates: 38 g, Fat: 12 g, Cholesterol: 59 mg, Fiber: 4.7 g, Sodium: 348 mg, Potassium: 653 mg, Phosphorus: 270 mg, Calcium: 133 mg

## Ingredients:

- 1 ½ cup of corn
- 2 cups of kidney beans (dried) soaked for 24 hours.
- 1 diced onion,
- 2 chicken breasts
- 1 can of tomatoes diced with green chilies.
- 1 teaspoon of cumin
- 3 tablespoons of ranch seasoning
- 1 teaspoon of onion powder
- 1 tablespoon of red chili powder
- 1 teaspoon of garlic powder
- 8-ounce package of cream cheese 1 packet

## Instructions:

Add chicken breast corn, onion beans, seasonings, canned tomatoes, and water to the slow cooker. Cover with cream cheese. Cook for 8 hours on low. Chicken is shredded when cooked. Stir it and serve.

## 242- Cauliflower Steaks

Preparation time: 5 minutes

Cooking Time: 35 minutes

Servings: 4

Difficulty Level: Easy

### Nutritional Information:

Calories: 119 kcal, protein: 2 g, carbohydrates: 6 g, Fat: 10 g, Cholesterol: 0 mg, Fiber: 2.3 g, Sodium: 106 mg, Potassium: 335 mg, Phosphorus: 50 mg, Calcium: 26 mg

### Ingredients:

- ¼ cup olive oil
- One large head cauliflower: sliced 4 'steaks.'
- 2 cloves garlic, minced.
- 1 tablespoon of fresh lemon juice
- Pinch of ground black or green pepper
- ½ teaspoon of red pepper flakes, or to taste.

### Instructions:

Preheat the oven to 400 degrees F. Lay parchment paper on the baking sheet. On the prepared and lined baking dish, put cauliflower steaks. Whisk ginger, black pepper, olive oil, red pepper flakes, and lemon juice together in a bowl. Coat the top surface of cauliflower steaks with this mixture. Bake for 15 minutes in the preheated oven. Flip them and pour the olive oil mixture on the steak. Roast for an extra 15 to 20 minutes until tender.

## 243- Slow Cooker Thai Chicken

Preparation time: 10 minutes

Cooking Time: 5-6 hours

Servings: 9

Difficulty Level: Easy

### Nutritional Information:

Calories: 159 kcal, protein: 23 g, carbohydrates: 1 g, Fat: 7 g, Cholesterol: 71 mg, Fiber: 0.2 g, Sodium: 64 mg, Potassium: 180 mg, Phosphorus: 132 mg, Calcium: 17 mg

### Ingredients:

- 7 tsp of Thai red curry paste
- 13 ½ ounces of coconut milk; unsweetened
- 1 tsp of garlic chopped.
- 1 head cauliflower uncooked, cut into florets.
- ½ tsp of ground ginger
- 2 medium carrots: ½ inch slices.
- 1 chopped sweet red pepper,
- 2 tbsp of sunflower seed butter (no salt)
- 1 pound of chicken breast, uncooked: 2-inch cubes.
- 1 fresh lime: six wedges.
- 3 medium sliced green onions.
- 1/3 cup of fresh cilantro, chopped.

### Instructions:

Coat chicken with 2 tsp of curry paste. Add coconut milk, ginger, 2-4 Tsp of curry paste, salt, and garlic in a slow cooker of 4 to 6 quarts in size. Add carrots, cauliflower, and red pepper. Add chicken to a mixture of vegetables. Cook for 5-6 hours on LOW until veggies are tender. Add sunflower seed butter and more curry paste into a slow cooker until combined well. Mix green onions and cilantro. Serve with a lime slice in a bowl.

## 244- Asparagus with Lemon Sauce

Preparation time: 5 minutes

Cooking Time: 20 minutes

Servings: 4

Difficulty Level: Easy

### Nutritional Information:

Calories: 59 kcal, protein: 2 g, carbohydrates: 6 g, Fat: 2 g, Cholesterol: 0 mg, Fiber: 3 g, Sodium: 2 mg, Potassium: 324 mg, Phosphorus: 64 mg, Calcium: 19 mg

### Ingredients:

- 1 fresh lemon (for peel and juice)
- 20 medium asparagus spears: trimmed.
- 1/8 teaspoon of ground black pepper
- 2 tablespoons of low-fat mayonnaise.

### Instructions:

Pour 1 inch of water into a 4-quart pot with a cover. Put asparagus in a steamer bucket and place it inside the pot. Cover and boil it over high heat. Lower the heat and cook until asparagus turns bright green and is easily stabbed with a knife; it will take 5-10 minutes. Do not overcook it. Add lemon zest, lemon juice, seasonings, and mayonnaise to a shallow bowl. Stir it and put it aside. Take off the pot from the heat once the asparagus gets tender and arrange them in a serving dish. Pour lemon sauce generously over the asparagus and serve it.

## 245- Vegetable Cutlets

Preparation time: 10 minutes

Cooking Time: 20 minutes

Servings: 6

Difficulty Level: Easy

### Nutritional Information:

Calories: 145 kcal, protein: 4 g, carbohydrates: 21 g, Fat: 5 g, Cholesterol: 0 mg, Fiber: 3.4 g, Sodium: 219 mg, Potassium: 241 mg, Phosphorus: 60 mg, Calcium: 75 mg

### Ingredients:

- 2 tablespoons of canola oil
- 1 cup of carrots
- 2 cups of green beans
- 1/4 teaspoon of salt
- 2 cups of cabbage
- 1/2 cup of white flour: all-purpose
- 1 teaspoon of red chili powder
- 1/2 teaspoon of lime juice
- 1 teaspoon of cumin powder
- 4 slices of white bread
- 1 teaspoon of cilantro powder
- 1/4 cup of fresh cilantro

### Instructions:

Wash, dry, and grate all vegetables (slice green beans). In water, soak the bread and drain it. Boil carrots and cabbage in a medium pan for 10 minutes. Then add green beans. Once vegetables are done, drain water and set them aside. Mix boiled vegetables with flour, seasonings, bread slices, lemon juice, and cilantro and blend them thoroughly. Make 12 patties. Heat oil in a saucepan over a low flame and add patties. Fry each side for 2-3 minutes until done. Serve them warm.

## 246- Southern Fried Okra

Preparation time: 5 minutes

Cooking Time: 30 minutes

Servings: 6

Difficulty Level: Easy

### Nutritional Information:

Calories: 213 kcal, protein: 5 g, carbohydrates: 20 g, Fat: 14 g, Cholesterol: 28 mg, Fiber: 3 g, Sodium: 67 mg, Potassium: 167 mg, Phosphorus: 79 mg, Calcium: 74 mg

### Ingredients:

- 1 medium egg
- ½ cup of unbleached flour
- 2 tablespoons of milk
- ½ cup of yellow cornmeal
- ¼ teaspoon of cayenne pepper
- 3 cups of okra, stems removed: ¼-inch pieces,
- ⅓ cup of sunflower oil
- ⅛ teaspoon of salt or to taste.
- ¼ teaspoon of black pepper, freshly ground.

### Instructions:

Set the oven to 300°F. Mix cornmeal, black pepper, flour, cayenne pepper, and salt in a medium dish with a whisk. In a separate shallow dish, beat milk and egg. Warm the sunflower oil in a wide skillet. Coat okra pieces with egg batter and then with cornmeal mixture. Fry them in a skillet and turn them after 2 minutes until golden. Use a slotted spoon to take them out from the oil. Drain on a paper towel. Transfer them to a baking dish and then to the oven. Once they are done, serve them hot.

## 247- Moroccan Couscous

Preparation time: 10 minutes

Cooking Time: 10 minutes

Servings: 5

Difficulty Level: Easy

### Nutritional Information:

Calories: 126 kcal, protein: 4 g, carbohydrates: 23 g, Fat: 2 g, Cholesterol: 0 mg, Fiber: 1.5 g, Sodium: 5.5 mg, Potassium: 57 mg, Phosphorus: 51 mg, Calcium: 10 mg

### Ingredients:

- ⅔ cup of dry couscous
- 2 tablespoons of chopped onion.
- 1 cup of water
- ½ tablespoon of margarine or olive oil

### Instructions:

Sauté the sliced onion in olive oil or margarine until soft. Boil water in a medium saucepan. Stir in the onion and couscous, and let it stand for 5 minutes. Fluff lightly before eating with a fork.

## 248- Lemon Rice with Vegetables

Preparation time: 5 minutes

Cooking Time: 30 minutes

Servings: 5

Difficulty Level: Easy

### Nutritional Information:

Calories: 183 kcal, protein: 3 g, carbohydrates: 27 g, Fat: 7 g, Cholesterol: 0 mg, Fiber: 0.7 g, Sodium: 13 mg, Potassium: 143 mg, Phosphorus: 37 mg, Calcium: 22 mg

### Ingredients:

- 3 tablespoons of unsalted margarine
- 1/4 cup of onion
- 1/2 cup of celery
- 1-1/4 cups of water
- 1-1/2 cups of fresh mushrooms
- 1/8 teaspoon of whole dried thyme
- 1 teaspoon of grated lemon zest
- 1/8 teaspoon of black pepper

- 2 tablespoons of lemon juice
- 10 tablespoons of rice, uncooked
- 1/8 teaspoon of herb seasoning

## Instructions:

Slash onion, mushrooms, and celery. Melt 1-1/2 tbsp of margarine in a large skillet and sauté onion and celery. Add seasonings, water, pepper, thyme, lemon zest, and juice. Cook it. Then add rice and cover it to boil on low heat for 20 minutes until rice is tender. In a shallow pan, melt 1-1/2 teaspoons of margarine and cook mushrooms until they're soft. Spread mushrooms over the mixture of rice and swirl to blend. Serve it warm.

## 249- Slow Cooker Chicken with Green Beans & Carrots

Preparation time:10minutes

Cooking Time:  3-6 hours

Servings: 4

Difficulty Level: Medium

## Nutritional Information:

Calories: 181 kcal, protein: 27 g, carbohydrates: 10 g, Fat: 3 g, Cholesterol: 70 mg, Fiber: 3.3 g, Sodium: 189 mg, Potassium: 431 mg, Phosphorus: 226mg, Calcium: 55 mg

## Ingredients:

- 1-1/2 cup frozen carrots, sliced
- 1-1/2 cup frozen Italian green beans
- 1/2 cup onion, diced
- 1-pound boneless, skinless chicken breasts
- 1/2 cup reduced-sodium chicken broth
- 2 teaspoons Worcestershire sauce
- 1 teaspoon of  herb seasoning blend

## Instructions:

Combine carrots, green beans, and onion. Place in a 4- or 6-quart slow cooker. Lay down the chicken breasts over the vegetables. Over the chicken, pour the broth. Add Worcestershire sauce and seasoning mix on top. Cook with a cover for 3 hours on high heat or 6 hours on low heat. Serve chicken breast with 3/4 cup vegetables and 2 tablespoons broth.

## 250- Fried Tofu with Dipping Sauce

Preparation time: 10 minutes

Cooking Time: 20 minutes

Servings: 2

Difficulty Level: Easy

## Nutritional Information:

Calories: 219 kcal, protein: 9 g, carbohydrates: 6 g, Fat: 19 g, Cholesterol: 0 mg, Fiber: 0.8 g, Sodium: 200 mg, Potassium: 176 mg, Phosphorus: 132 mg, Calcium: 160 mg

## Ingredients:

- 6 ounces of firm tofu
- 1 garlic clove
- 2 tablespoons of vegetable oil
- 1-1/2 teaspoons of sesame oil
- 1 teaspoon of sugar
- 2 teaspoons of low-sodium soy sauce.
- 1 green onion
- 1 teaspoon of hot pepper flakes

## Instructions:

Split Tofu into four rectangular pieces with a paper towel and dry each piece. Heat two teaspoons of vegetable oil on high flame in a frying pan. Cook tofu for 5 to 7 minutes or until golden brown on low-medium heat. Flip it over and cook for 5 to 7 minutes until the bottom of each section is golden brown. In a shallow mixing bowl, dipping sauce combines chopped green onion, minced garlic, honey or sugar, low-sodium soy sauce, hot pepper flakes, and sesame oil and serve with Tofu.

# 251- Roasted Beet Noodles With Baby Kale and Pesto

Preparation time: 5 minutes

Cooking Time: 20 minutes

Servings: 3

Difficulty Level: Easy

## Nutritional Information:

Calories: 263 kcal, protein: 3 g, carbohydrates: 10 g, Fat: 25 g, Cholesterol: 0 mg, Fiber: 3 g, Sodium: 55 mg, Potassium: 182 mg, Phosphorus: 226mg, Calcium: 20 mg

## Ingredients:

- 2 cups of baby kale
- olive oil as cooking spray
- 2 media peeled, beets, Blade C noodles trimmed.

**For the pesto:**

- 1/2 cup of peanuts
- 3 cup basil leaves, packed.
- 1/2 teaspoon of ground sea salt
- 1/4 cup of olive oil
- 1 large, minced clove of garlic,
- 1/4 teaspoon of ground pepper

## Instructions:

Preheat an oven to 425 degrees Fahrenheit. Spread the beet noodles on a baking sheet, coated with cooking spray, and season with pepper and salt. Bake for 5-10 minutes, until beets are al dente, or until done to your liking.

While the noodles are cooking, put all the pesto ingredients in a food blender and blend until smooth. Taste and make any necessary adjustments. Toss the beets with the pesto and greens after they've been cooked. Serve.

# 252- White sea bass and dill relish

Preparation time: 10 minutes

Cooking Time: 20 minutes

Servings: 4

Difficulty Level: Easy

## Nutritional Information:

Calories: 115 kcal, protein: 22 g, carbohydrates: 1 g, Fat: 2 g, Cholesterol: 46 mg, Fiber: 0.2 g, Sodium: 127 mg, Potassium: 138 mg, Phosphorus: 204 mg, Calcium: 15.46 mg

## Ingredients:

- 1 teaspoon of pickled drained baby capers,
- 1 lemon, quarters
- 1 1/2 tablespoons of chopped white onion.
- 1 teaspoon of lemon juice
- 1 1/2 teaspoons of fresh dill; chopped.
- 4 fillets of white sea bass, 4 ounces each
- 1 teaspoon of Dijon mustard

## Instructions:

Preheat an oven to 375 degrees Fahrenheit. Combine the mustard, capers, onion, dill, and lemon juice in a small bowl. Stir it well. Each fillet should be placed on a piece of aluminum foil. Squeeze one lemon wedge over each fillet, and 1/4 of dill relish is distributed over each piece. Wrap the aluminum foil around the fish and bake for 10 to 12 minutes, or until the fish is white throughout when checked with the tip of a knife. Serve right away.

## 253- Cilantro Lime Cauliflower "Rice"

Preparation time: 5 minutes

Cooking Time:  20 minutes

Servings: 4

Difficulty Level: Easy

### Nutritional Information:

Calories: 93 kcal, protein: 3.1 g, carbohydrates: 9.6 g, Fat: 6 g, Cholesterol: 15.3 mg, Fiber: 4 g, Sodium: 87.1 mg, Potassium: 484.3 mg, Phosphorus: 226 mg, Calcium: 40 mg

### Ingredients:

- 1 tablespoon of water
- 1 head of cauliflower, slashed into florets.
- 1 lime, juiced & zested.
- 2 tablespoons of butter (Optional)
- ½ cup of chopped cilantro

### Instructions:

Shred cauliflower florets or process them until they resemble rice in a food processor. In a covered microwave-safe dish, combine grated cauliflower and water. Cook cauliflower in the microwave on high for 7 minutes, or until tender. Toss cooked cauliflower with cilantro, lime juice, zest,  and butter until thoroughly combined.

## 254- Salmon Skewers

Preparation time: 30 minutes

Cooking Time:  30 minutes

Servings: 2

Difficulty Level: Easy

### Nutritional Information:

Calories: 561 kcal, protein: 30 g, carbohydrates: 7.8 g, Fat: 43.2 g, Cholesterol: 82.7 mg, Fiber: 1 g, Sodium: 87.4 mg, Potassium: 656.2 mg, Phosphorus: 324 mg, Calcium: 20 mg

### Ingredients:

- ⅓ cup of lemon juice
- 2 skinless salmon fillets (6 ounces), 1-inch thick, 2-inch-long strips
- 1 tablespoon of fresh dill; chopped.
- ¼ cup of white wine
- 1 tablespoon of fresh mint; chopped.
- 1 pinch of red pepper flakes; crushed.
- 2 tablespoons of fresh parsley; chopped.
- ¼ cup of olive oil
- 2 tablespoons of minced garlic

### Instructions:

Preheat the grill to medium-low. In the base of a baking dish, place the salmon. Mix the mint, wine, lemon juice,  dill, garlic, parsley, and red pepper flakes in a mixing bowl. Slowly pour in olive oil while stirring thoroughly. Over the fish, pour the mixture. Refrigerate the salmon for 30 minutes after it has been marinated. Thread the fish lengthwise onto metal or moist wooden skewers. Cook over a hot grill until the center is opaque, approximately 4 minutes on each side. Serve right away.

## 255- Grilled Basil Chicken and Tomatoes

Preparation time: 5 minutes

Cooking Time:  25 minutes

Servings: 4

Difficulty Level: Easy

## Nutritional Information:

Calories: 177 kcal, protein: 24 g, carbohydrates: 6.3 g, Fat: 5 g, Cholesterol: 63 mg, Fiber: 1 g, Sodium: 171 mg, Potassium: 585.5 mg, Phosphorus:210 mg, Calcium: 14 mg

## Ingredients:

- 2 tablespoons of olive oil
- 1/4 cup of fresh basil leaves; tightly packed
- 3/4 cup of balsamic vinegar
- 1/2 teaspoon of salt
- 1 minced garlic clove,
- 4 skinless, boneless chicken breast halves (4 ounces each)
- 8 plum tomatoes

## Instructions:

In a blender, combine the first five ingredients for the marinade. Four tomatoes are quartered, added to a blender, covered, and mixed until smooth. To grill the remaining tomatoes, cut them in half.

Combine the 2/3 cup of marinade and chicken in a bowl; refrigerate for 1 hour, flipping periodically. Save the rest of the marinade for serving.

Drain the chicken and toss out the marinade. Place the chicken on a grill rack that has been greased over medium heat. Cover and grill chicken for 4-6 minutes on each side, or until a thermometer reads 165°F. Cover and grill tomatoes for 2-4 minutes on each side over medium heat, until gently browned. Serve the chicken and tomatoes with the marinade that was saved.

## 256- Chicken Veggie Packets

Preparation time: 5 minutes

Cooking Time: 25 minutes

Servings: 4

Difficulty Level: Easy

## Nutritional Information:

Calories: 175 kcal, protein: 25 g, carbohydrates: 11 g, Fat: 3 g, Cholesterol: 63 mg, Fiber: 4 g, Sodium: 100 mg, Potassium: 463 mg, Phosphorus: 365 mg, Calcium: 46 mg

## Ingredients:

- 1/2 pound of fresh sliced mushrooms
- 4 skinless, boneless chicken breast halves (4 ounces each)
- 1-1/2 cups of fresh baby carrots
- 1/4 teaspoon of pepper
- 1 cup of pearl onions
- 3 teaspoons of minced fresh thyme
- 1/2 cup of sweet red pepper; julienned
- Lemon wedges, optional
- 1/2 teaspoon of salt, optional

## Instructions:

Preheat the oven to 375 degrees Fahrenheit. Flatten the chicken breasts to 1/2-inch thickness and put on a heavy-duty foil sheet (about 12 in. square). Over the chicken, layer the mushrooms, onions, carrots, and red pepper, season with thyme, pepper, and salt, if preferred.

Seal the foil firmly around the chicken and veggies. Place on a baking tray. Cook for approximately 20 minutes, or until the chicken juices flow clear. Serve with lemon wedges if preferred.

## 257- Avocado, Tomato & Chicken Sandwich

Preparation time: 10 minutes

Cooking Time: 15 minutes

Servings: 1

Difficulty Level: Easy

## Nutritional Information:

Calories: 347 kcal, protein: 31.2 g, carbohydrates: 28.4 g, Fat: 12.3 g, Cholesterol: 62.7 mg, Fiber: 4 g, Sodium: 258.2 mg, Potassium: 646.8 mg, Phosphorus: 464.5 mg, Calcium: 60 mg

## Ingredients:

- ¼ ripe avocado
- 2 slices of multigrain bread
- 2 slices of tomato
- 3 ounces of cooked skinless, boneless chicken breast, sliced.

## Instructions:

Bread should be toasted. With a fork, mash the avocado and put it over one slice of bread. Add the chicken, tomato, and the second slice of bread to the top. You can poach chicken in a recipe if you don't have the cooked chicken. In a skillet or saucepan, place skinless, boneless chicken breasts. Cover with lightly salted water and boil it. Cover, lower heat to a low simmer, and cook until the center is no longer pink, for about 10 to 15 minutes, depending on the size.

## 258- Italian Chicken and Penne

Preparation time: 5 minutes

Cooking Time: 30 minutes

Servings: 6

Difficulty Level: Easy

## Nutritional Information:

Calories: 291 kcal, protein: 23 g, carbohydrates: 34 g, Fat: 7 g, Cholesterol: 46 mg, Fiber: 3 g, Sodium: 214 mg, Potassium: 196.4 mg, Phosphorus: 245 mg, Calcium: 80 mg

## Ingredients:

- 1-pound skinless, boneless chicken breasts, 1/2-inch pieces
- 8 ounces of penne pasta; uncooked
- 1 small julienned green pepper,
- 1 minced garlic clove,
- 1/2 cup of chopped onion
- 1/2 teaspoon of Italian seasoning
- 1 tablespoon of olive oil
- 1 cup of halved grape or cherry tomatoes
- 1 cup of fresh mushrooms; sliced.
- 1/3 cup of part-skim shredded mozzarella cheese
- 1 can of pizza sauce; (8 ounces)

## Instructions:

Drain pasta after cooking according to package instructions. Stir-fry the onion, pepper, chicken, and garlic in oil in a nonstick pan until the chicken is no longer pink. Heat through the mushrooms, pasta, sauce, tomatoes, and seasoning. Remove the pan from the heat. Sprinkle with cheese and set aside to melt.

## 259- Chicken and Mint Coleslaw Wraps

Preparation time: 10 minutes

Cooking Time: 20 minutes

Servings: 6

Difficulty Level: Easy

## Nutritional Information:

Calories: 304 kcal, protein: 32.6 g, carbohydrates: 31.2 g, Fat: 6.1 g, Cholesterol: 71 mg, Fiber: 2.6 g, Sodium: 121 mg, Potassium: 183.9 mg, Phosphorus: 200 mg, Calcium: 25.6 mg

## Ingredients:

- ⅛ teaspoon of salt

- 4 (6-ounce) boneless skinless chicken breast halves
- ⅓ cup of fresh lemon juice
- Cooking spray
- 2 teaspoons of sugar
- 1 tablespoon of fresh ginger; bottled ground
- 3 cups of angel hair coleslaw
- ¼ teaspoon of red pepper; crushed.
- ½ cup of chopped fresh mint.
- 6 flour tortillas(8-inch)
- 1 poblano chili, seeded, halved lengthwise, and thinly sliced.

## Instructions:

Using a meat mallet or rolling pin, pound each chicken breast half to 1/4-inch thickness between two sheets of heavy-duty plastic wrap. Season chicken with salt and pepper. Over medium-high heat, place a coated with cooking spray wide nonstick skillet. Add the chicken and cook for 4 1/2 minutes for each side, or until cooked through. Cut the chicken into small strips on a chopping board. Mix the juice, sugar, ginger, and red pepper in a large bowl. Toss in the chicken strips, mint, coleslaw, and chili to coat thoroughly. Toasted tortillas should be warmed according to the package instructions. Distribute the chicken mixture equally among the tortillas and wrap them up. Each rolled tortilla should be cut in half crosswise.

## 260- Three Sisters Soup

Preparation time: 5 minutes

Cooking Time: 30 minutes

Servings: 6

Difficulty Level: Easy

## Nutritional Information:

Calories: 145 kcal, protein: 9 g, carbohydrates: 28 g, Fat: 1 g, Cholesterol: 0 mg, Fiber: 5 g, Sodium: 87 mg, Potassium: 74.7 mg, Phosphorus: 58.7 mg, Calcium: 61 mg

## Ingredients:

- 16 oz. Low-sodium canned yellow corn or hominy drained and rinsed.
- 6 cups of low-sodium fat-free, chicken or vegetable stock
- 1/2 tsp. of curry powder
- 16 oz. low-sodium canned kidney beans (drained, rinsed)
- 15 oz. of cooked, canned pumpkin
- 1 small chopped onion.
- 5 fresh sage leaves OR 1/2 tsp. of dried sage
- 1 chopped rib celery

## Instructions:

Bring the chicken stock to a boil. Corn/hominy, onion, beans, and celery are added. Boil for 10 minutes at a low temperature. Simmer for 20 minutes over medium-low heat with curry, sage leaves, and pumpkin.

# CHAPTER 9

## Sauces, Dressings & Seasonings

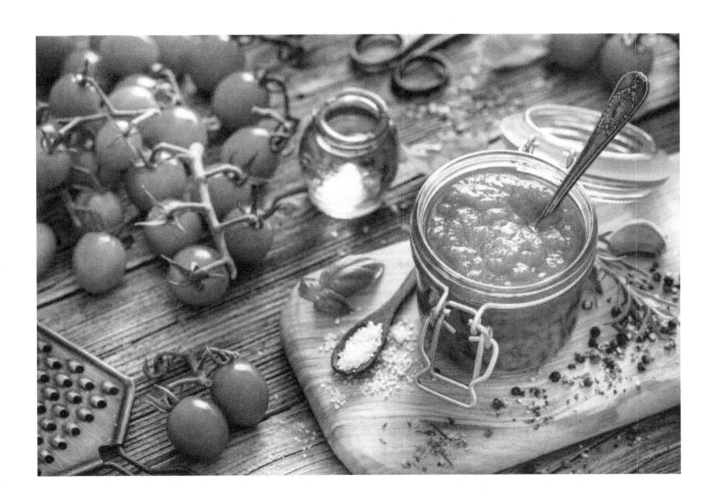

# 261- Low Salt Ketchup

Preparation time: 10 minutes

Cooking Time: 40 minutes

Servings: 64

Difficulty Level: Easy

## Nutritional Information:

Calories: 12 kcal, protein: 0 g, carbohydrates: 3 g, Fat: 0 g, Cholesterol: 0 mg, Fiber: 2 g, Sodium: 17 mg, Potassium: 62 mg, Phosphorus: 1 mg, Calcium: 1 mg

## Ingredients:

- 1/2 cup of cider vinegar
- 3/4 cup of onion, chopped.
- 1/3 cup of Sugar
- 2 tsp of dry mustard
- 1 tbsp molasses
- 1/4 tsp ground cinnamon
- 1/2 tsp celery seed
- 1/4 tsp dried basil
- 2 (6-oz.) can tomato paste.
- 1/4 tsp cloves
- 1 cup of water
- 1/4 tsp dried tarragon
- 1 clove of garlic, minced.
- 1/4 tsp pepper

## Instructions:

Put all ingredients except water and tomato paste in a blender or food processor, and blend until smooth. In a Dutch oven or large saucepan, pour the mixture. Add 3 cups of water and two 6-oz tomato paste cans. Simmer, uncovered, for around 35 minutes or until the mixture has decreased to half the initial volume; stir regularly. Pour into jars and place for up to 1 month in the refrigerator or freezer for up to 10 months.

# 262- Homemade BBQ Sauce

Preparation time: 0 minutes

Cooking Time: 10 minutes

Servings: 16

Difficulty Level: Easy

## Nutritional Information:

Calories: 55 kcal, protein: 0 g, carbohydrates: 7 g, Fat: 1 g, Cholesterol: 3 mg, Fiber: 0.2 g, Sodium: 51 mg, Potassium: 32 mg, Phosphorus: 5 mg, Calcium: 5 mg

## Ingredients:

- 1/4 cup of honey
- 2 tbsp of canola oil
- 2 tbsp of Brown Sugar
- 2 tbsp of sweet onion
- 1/4 cup of apple cider vinegar
- 1 small garlic clove
- 1 cup of water
- 2 tbsp of tomato paste
- 1 tsp of browning and seasoning sauce
- 2 tsp of dry mustard
- 1 tsp of hot pepper sauce
- 1/4 tsp of salt
- 1-1/2 tbsp of butter

## Instructions:

Mince a clove of garlic and grate the onion. Cook all the ingredients until the butter is melted and the onion and garlic are lightly cooked over low heat. The sauce is ready for usage or kept for up to one week in a sealed jar in the refrigerator.

# 263- Sweet Chili Thai Sauce

Preparation time: 2 minutes

Cooking Time: 10 minutes

Servings: 8

Difficulty Level: Easy

## Nutritional Information:

Calories: 54 kcal, protein: 0 g, carbohydrates: 14 g, Fat: 0 g, Cholesterol: 0 mg, Fiber: 0.1 g, Sodium: 68 mg, Potassium: 14 mg, Phosphorus: 3 mg, Calcium: 3 mg

## Ingredients:

- ¾ cup of cider vinegar
- 1 cup of water
- ½ cup of Sugar
- 1 tsp of minced garlic
- 2 tsp of ketchup
- 1 tsp of ginger
- 4 tsp of cornstarch
- 2 tsp of red pepper flakes

## Instructions:

Boil water and cider vinegar. Add ginger, sugar, garlic, ketchup, and red pepper flakes, mix and boil for 5 minutes. Add cornstarch by sifting and stirring constantly. For the thick sauce, add more corn starch.

## 264- All-Purpose No-Salt Seasoning Mix

Preparation time: 5 minutes

Cooking Time: 0 minutes

Servings: 10

Difficulty Level: Easy

## Nutritional Information:

Calories: 20.7 kcal, protein: 1 g, carbohydrates: 3.7 g, Fat: 1 g, Cholesterol: 0 mg, Fiber: 1.2 g, Sodium: 3.2 mg, Potassium: 23.9 mg, Phosphorus: 80.45 mg, Calcium: 4 mg

## Ingredients:

- 1 ¼ teaspoon ground thyme
- 1 teaspoon ground mace

- 1 tablespoon garlic powder
- 1 ½ teaspoon dried parsley
- 1 ½ teaspoon dried basil
- 1 teaspoon ground black pepper
- 1 teaspoon onion powder
- 1 ¼ teaspoon dried savory
- ¼ teaspoon cayenne pepper
- 1 teaspoon dried sage

## Instructions:

In a bowl, mix basil, garlic powder, parsley, thyme, savory, onion powder, mace, sage, cayenne pepper, and black Pepper, and reserve it in a covered jar.

## 265- Garlic-Herb Seasoning

Preparation time: 5 minutes

Cooking Time: 0 minutes

Servings: 6

Difficulty Level: Easy

## Nutritional Information:

Calories: 5.2 kcal, protein: 0.2 g, carbohydrates: 1 g, Fat: 0.2 g, Cholesterol: 0 mg, Fiber: 0.4 g, Sodium: 0.8 mg, Potassium: 20 mg, Phosphorus: 7 mg, Calcium: 2 mg

## Ingredients:

- 1 tsp Powdered lemon rind
- 2 tsp Garlic powder
- 1 tsp Oregano
- 1 tsp Basil

## Instructions:

In a processor, combine ingredients. Store rice grains to avoid clumping in a sealed jar.

## 266- Salt-free Cajun Seasoning

Preparation time: 5 minutes

Cooking Time: 0 minutes

Servings: 20

Difficulty Level: Easy

## Nutritional Information:

Calories: 6 kcal, protein: 0 g, carbohydrates: 1 g, Fat: 0 g, Cholesterol: 0 mg, Fiber: 0.5 g, Sodium: 1 mg, Potassium: 34 mg, Phosphorus: 7 mg, Calcium: 8 mg

## Ingredients:

- 1 tbsp garlic powder
- 2 tbsp paprika
- 2 tsp black pepper
- 2 tsp dried oregano
- 2 tsp cayenne pepper
- 1 tbsp of onion powder
- 2 tsp dried thyme

## Instructions:

Combine all ingredients in a bowl and store it in an airtight jar. Use it when required.

## 267- Simple Low Sodium Soy Sauce

Preparation time: 5 minutes

Cooking Time: 5 minutes

Servings: 32

Difficulty Level: Easy

## Nutritional Information:

Calories: 10 kcal, protein: 0 g, carbohydrates: 2 g, Fat: 0 g, Cholesterol: 0 mg, Fiber: 0 g, Sodium: 38 mg, Potassium: 113 mg, Phosphorus: 3 mg, Calcium: 2 mg

## Ingredients:

- 2 garlic cloves
- 3/4 cup of vinegar

- 1 tbsp onion powder
- 3 tbsp dark molasses

## Instructions:

Heat the vinegar until it is warm, but do not boil it. Peel and dice the garlic cloves and add them to the hot vinegar. In the refrigerator, place it covered to set overnight. Strain the garlic and discard it. Mix the garlic vinegar with the onion powder and molasses in a glass jar and place it in the refrigerator. Shake it before using it and use hot. It lasts around 1 month.

## 268- Red Chili Mustard Vinegar

Preparation time: 5 minutes

Cooking Time: 0 minutes

Servings: 8

Difficulty Level: Easy

## Nutritional Information:

Calories: 134 kcal, protein: 1 g, carbohydrates: 2 g, Fat: 1 g, Cholesterol: 0 mg, Fiber: 2 g, Sodium: 40 mg, Potassium: 31 mg, Phosphorus: 4 mg, Calcium: 4 mg

## Ingredients:

- 1 tbsp shallots, chopped.
- 2 tbsp Dijon mustard
- 1/2 cup of olive oil
- Pepper to taste
- 1/4 cup of vinegar
- 1 tbsp of chili powder

## Instructions:

Mix shallots, chili powder, vinegar, mustard, and Pepper. Whisk in the oil slowly until it is mixed. Taste and add chili powder or spice if required.

## 269- Poultry Seasoning

Preparation time: 5 minutes

Cooking Time: 0 minutes

Servings: 11

Difficulty Level: Easy

## Nutritional Information:

Calories: 3 kcal, protein: 0 g, carbohydrates: 0 g, Fat: 0 g, Cholesterol: 0 mg, Fiber: 0 g, Sodium: 0 mg, Potassium: 8 mg, Phosphorus: 1 mg, Calcium: 1 mg

## Ingredients:

- 1 tsp black pepper: ground
- 2 tbsp ground sage: dried
- 2 tsp dried marjoram
- 2 tsp dried thyme

## Instructions:

In a small bowl, combine all ingredients. Add this blend to an airtight jar. Good to use for one year.

## 270- Mexican Seasoning

Preparation time: 5 minutes

Cooking Time: 0 minutes

Servings: 8

Difficulty Level: Easy

## Nutritional Information:

Calories: 8 kcal, protein: 0 g, carbohydrates: 2 g, Fat: 0 g, Cholesterol: 0 mg, Fiber: 0.7 g, Sodium: 30 mg, Potassium: 38 mg, Phosphorus: 7 mg, Calcium: 9 mg

## Ingredients:

- 2 tsp paprika
- 3 tsp chili powder
- 2 tsp ground cumin
- 1/2 tsp garlic powder
- 1/8 tsp cayenne pepper

- 1 tsp of onion powder

## Instructions:

Mix the spices in a small container or a bowl. Preserve it for up to 6 months of preservation in a sealed jar. Season meat or vegetables.

## 271- Easy Gravy

Preparation time: 5 minutes

Cooking Time: 5 minutes

Servings: 8

Difficulty Level: Easy

## Nutritional Information:

Calories: 85 kcal, protein: 2 g, carbohydrates: 4 g, Fat: 11 g, Cholesterol: 2 mg, Fiber: 0.1 g, Sodium: 150 mg, Potassium: 58 mg, Phosphorus: 24 mg, Calcium: 5 mg

## Ingredients:

- 1/2 tsp of Black Pepper
- 2 cups of low sodium chicken or beef broth
- 1/2 tsp of paprika
- 1/3 cup of corn starch
- 1/2 tsp of onion powder
- 1/2 tsp of garlic powder

## Instructions:

Mix all the ingredients until no lumps and place them into a saucepan. Cook, stirring regularly, over medium heat until thickened. For 2 minutes, boil slowly and serve over rice, pasta, beef, etc.

## 272- Fajita Flavor Marinade

Preparation time: 5 minutes

Cooking Time: 0 minutes

Servings: 15

Difficulty Level: Easy

## Nutritional Information:

Calories: 33 kcal, protein: 0 g, carbohydrates: 2 g, Fat: 1 g, Cholesterol: 0 mg, Fiber: 0.5 g, Sodium: 0 mg, Potassium: 42 mg, Phosphorus: 5 mg, Calcium: 6 mg

## Ingredients:

- 3 tbsp vegetable oil
- juice from 2 limes
- 1 jalapeño finely diced.
- juice from 1 orange
- 2 crushed cloves of garlic or 1/4 teaspoon dried.
- Juice from 1 grapefruit

## Instructions:

In a small bowl, mix all ingredients. Coat vegetables or meat with it. Marinate for 1 hour before grilling, barbequing, or pan-frying.

## 273- Alfredo Sauce

Preparation time: 5 minutes

Cooking Time: 20 minutes

Servings: 8

Difficulty Level: Easy

## Nutritional Information:

Calories: 124 kcal, protein: 3 g, carbohydrates: 3 g, Fat: 12 g, Cholesterol: 36 mg, Fiber: 0 g, Sodium: 153 mg, Potassium: 65 mg, Phosphorus: 70 mg, Calcium: 87 mg

## Ingredients:

- 3 tbsp of all-purpose flour
- 1/4 cup of olive oil
- 1 clove of garlic, minced.

- 4 ounces cream cheese
- 2 cups of rice milk
- 1/3 cup Parmesan cheese: shredded
- 1 tbsp lemon juice
- 1/4 tsp ground nutmeg

## Instructions:

Over medium heat, heat the olive oil in a large pan. To make a paste, add flour, whisk, and chopped garlic. Then add rice milk slowly, whisking regularly to avoid lumps. Let the mixture simmer and let it thicken. Add cream cheese and blend thoroughly. Take it off from the heat. Add 1/3 cup of Parmesan cheese, lemon juice, and nutmeg. Mix thoroughly. Serve over pasta, steamed vegetables, chicken, etc.

## 274 Basil Oil

Preparation time: 20 minutes

Cooking Time: 10 minutes

Servings: 16

Difficulty Level: Easy

## Nutritional Information:

Calories: 135 kcal, protein: 0 g, carbohydrates: 0 g, Fat: 1 g, Cholesterol: 0 mg, Fiber: 15 g, Sodium: 0 mg, Potassium: 5 mg, Phosphorus: 0 mg, Calcium: 1 mg

## Ingredients:

- 1 cup olive oil or vegetable oil
- 1 1/2 cups of basil leaves: fresh

## Instructions:

Rinse 1 1/2 cups of finely packed fresh basil leaves and drain them. Pat leaves for drying them. Stir the basil leaves and 1 cup of olive oil or vegetable oil in a blender or food processor. Just whirl until the leaves are finely sliced (do not puree).

Over medium heat, pours the mixture into a 1 to 1 1/2-quart pan. Stir regularly for 3-4 minutes until oil spills along the pan's edges and the temperature reaches 165 degrees F. To disable any bacteria in the mixture, ensure the oil is hot to this temperature. Remove from heat and allow it to stay for around an hour before it cools. Line a fine wire strainer placed over a wide bowl with two layers of cheesecloth.

Pour a combination of oil into a strainer. Gently press the basil onto the remaining oil until after the oil moves through. Serve the oil or hold it in the refrigerator in an airtight jar for up to 3 months. When cooled, the olive oil will solidify but liquefy rapidly when it returns to room temperature.

## 275- BBQ Rub Chicken

Preparation time: 5 minutes

Cooking Time:  0 minutes

Servings: 4

Difficulty Level: Easy

### Nutritional Information:

Calories: 20  kcal, protein: 0 g, carbohydrates: 4 g, Fat: 1 g, Cholesterol: 0 mg, Fiber: 0 g, Sodium: 9 mg, Potassium: 34 mg, Phosphorus: 7 mg, Calcium: 6 mg

### Ingredients:

- 1/8 tsp red pepper: ground (optional)
- 1 tbsp Brown Sugar
- 1 tsp chili powder
- 1 tsp smoked paprika.
- 1/8 tsp allspice
- 1 teaspoon of onion powder
- 1 tsp garlic, granulated.
- 1/4 tsp mustard powder
- 1 tsp cumin

### Instructions:

Mix all ingredients in a bowl thoroughly. Before cooking, coat on chicken or meat Rub.

## 276- Chinese Five-Spice Blend

Preparation time: 5 minutes

Cooking Time:  0 minutes

Servings: 22

Difficulty Level: Easy

### Nutritional Information:

Calories: 20  kcal, protein: 0 g, carbohydrates: 4 g, Fat: 1 g, Cholesterol: 0 mg, Fiber: 1 g, Sodium: 14 mg, Potassium: 49 mg, Phosphorus: 4 mg, Calcium: 1 mg

### Ingredients:

- 2 tbsp cinnamon: ground
- 1 tsp of ground allspice
- 1/4 cup of ginger
- 1 tsp anise seed
- 2 tsp ground cloves

### Instructions:

Combine all ingredients in a bowl and store it in an airtight jar. Whole spices can be used for 2 years and ground spices for one year.

## 277- Simple Soup Base

Preparation time: 5 minutes

Cooking Time:  10 minutes

Servings: 6

Difficulty Level: Easy

### Nutritional Information:

Calories: 98  kcal, protein: 4.12 g, carbohydrates: 12 g, Fat: 4 g, Cholesterol: 0 mg, Fiber: 2.1 g,

Sodium: 38.2 mg, Potassium: 7 mg, Phosphorus: 5 mg, Calcium: 8 mg

## Ingredients:

- 1/4 tsp dry mustard
- 2 tbsp flour
- 1/4 tsp paprika
- 2 tbsp margarine or butter
- 1/2 tsp each parsley, basil, or any other herbs
- 2 cups of milk

## Instructions:

In a 2-cup glass measuring cup, mix margarine or butter and flour. For 30 seconds, microwave it, stir, and microwave for an additional 30 seconds. Add spices, milk, and microwave for 1 minute, then stir again. Microwave for another 1 minute if it's not thickened. Instead of creamed soups, use them. Add the sautéed mushrooms to the mushroom soup. Sauteed celery is added to the celery cream. To create chicken cream, add the fried, diced chicken.

## 278- Honey Dressing

Preparation time: 5 minutes

Cooking Time: 0 minutes

Servings: 7

Difficulty Level: Easy

## Nutritional Information:

Calories: 97 kcal, protein: 0 g, carbohydrates: 11 g, Fat: 6 g, Cholesterol: 0 mg, Fiber: 0 g, Sodium: 178 mg, Potassium: 24 mg, Phosphorus: 4 mg, Calcium: 1 mg

## Ingredients:

- 1 tsp of dried mustard
- ½ cup of Sugar
- 1 tsp of paprika

- ¼ cup of vinegar
- 1 cup of canola oil
- ½ cup of honey
- 1 tsp of onion, grated.
- 2 Tbsp of lemon juice

## Instructions:

Combine dry ingredients, then add vinegar, honey, onion, and lemon juice. In a food processor or blender, blend and add oil gradually.

## 279- Coleslaw Dressing

Preparation time: 5 minutes

Cooking Time: 0 minutes

Servings: 6

Difficulty Level: Easy

## Nutritional Information:

Calories: 55.9 kcal, protein: 0 g, carbohydrates: 6.8 g, Fat: 3.4 g, Cholesterol: 4.3 mg, Fiber: 0.1 g, Sodium: 272 mg, Potassium: 8.5 mg, Phosphorus: 5.1 mg, Calcium: 6.1 mg

## Ingredients:

- 1/2 cup of Mayonnaise
- 1/4 cup of Vinegar
- Salt and Pepper to taste
- 1/4 cup of Sugar

## Instructions:

In a small bowl, mix all ingredients thoroughly. This Dressing can be used with cabbage.

## 280- Italian Seasoning

Preparation time: 5 minutes

Cooking Time: 0 minutes

Servings: 6

Difficulty Level: Easy

## Nutritional Information:

Calories: 17.5 kcal, protein: 0.8 g, carbohydrates: 3.9 g, Fat: 0.3 g, Cholesterol: 0 mg, Fiber: 1.7 g, Sodium: 3.4 mg, Potassium: 85.6 mg, Phosphorus: 16.90 mg, Calcium: 6 mg

## Ingredients:

- 1 Tbsp of Garlic Powder
- 1/4 tsp of Black Pepper
- 3 Tbsp of Oregano
- 1 tsp of Parsley
- 2 tsp of Onion Powder
- 3 Tbsp of Basil

## Instructions:

Combine oregano, basil, garlic powder, onion powder, parsley, and black Pepper. Store it in an airtight jar.

## 281- Low-Sodium Mayonnaise

Preparation time: 10 minutes

Cooking Time: 0 minutes

Servings: 3 cups

Difficulty Level: Easy

## Nutritional Information:

Calories: 83 kcal, protein: 0 g, carbohydrates: 0 g, Fat: 9 g, Cholesterol: 9 mg, Fiber: 0 g, Sodium: 2 mg, Potassium: 3 mg, Phosphorus: 2 mg, Calcium: 1 mg

## Ingredients:

- 1/2 tsp of black pepper
- 2 tsp of ground mustard
- 1/2 tsp of paprika
- 2 large eggs (pasteurized)
- 1-2 cups of canola oil
- 2-3 Tbsp of apple cider vinegar

- 1/2 tsp of garlic powder

## Instructions:

In the mixer, add spices, eggs, and vinegar. Run the blender at its slowest level until it's well blended. Until the mayonnaise thickens, keep the blender running and gradually add the canola oil, increasing the blender's speed. Store it in the refrigerator.

## 282- White Bread Dressing

Preparation time: 5 minutes

Cooking Time: 30-35 minutes

Servings: 12

Difficulty Level: Easy

## Nutritional Information:

Calories: 241 kcal, protein: 5 g, carbohydrates: 17 g, Fat: 17 g, Cholesterol: 41 mg, Fiber: 2 g, Sodium: 184 mg, Potassium: 122 mg, Phosphorus: 64 mg, Calcium: 71 mg

## Ingredients:

- ¼ cup of chopped onions.
- 2 tbsp of margarine
- 1 ½ cups of breadcrumbs or 3 slices of bread crumbled.
- ¼ cup of unsalted chicken broth
- 1 tsp of poultry seasoning.
- ¼ cup of chopped celery.
- ¼ tsp of garlic powder

## Instructions:

In a shallow pan, heat the margarine and add onions. Stir until you have tender onions. Add breadcrumbs and continuously stir them to avoid blistering. Take it off from the heat. Add the celery, seasoning of the meat, chicken broth, and garlic powder. Mix thoroughly. Pour it into a small baking pan. Bake at 375°F for 30 minutes. If the Dressing is too dry, add water if required.

# 283- Non-dairy Cheesy Sauce

Preparation time: 5 minutes

Cooking Time: 10 minutes

Servings: 16

Difficulty Level: Easy

## Nutritional Information:

Calories: 21 kcal, protein: 1 g, carbohydrates: 4 g, Fat: 0 g, Cholesterol: 0 mg, Fiber: 0.5 g, Sodium: 1 mg, Potassium: 39 mg, Phosphorus: 22 mg, Calcium: 2 mg

## Ingredients:

- 1 cup of water
- 1/2 cup of nutritional yeast
- 1 tsp of turmeric
- 1/2 tsp of onion powder
- 1/2 cup of all-purpose flour
- 1/2 tsp of garlic powder

## Instructions:

Place all the dry ingredients in a pot, whisk to mix, and add the water. Stir periodically over medium-high heat until the sauce meets the ideal thickness. Take it off from the heat and serve.

# 284 Roasted Red Pepper Tomato Sauce

Preparation time: 15 minutes

Cooking Time: 3 minutes

Servings: 4

Difficulty Level: Easy

## Nutritional Information:

Calories: 75 kcal, protein: 1 g, carbohydrates: 3 g, Fat: 7 g, Cholesterol: 0 mg, Fiber: 0.8 g, Sodium: 82 mg, Potassium: 148 mg, Phosphorus: 18 mg, Calcium: 17 mg

## Ingredients:

- 1 garlic clove
- 1/2 cup of red peppers: roasted.
- 2 tbsp of olive oil
- 1/2 cup of tomato sauce: low-sodium
- 1/4 tsp of red pepper chili flakes
- 1 tsp of dried Italian seasoning

## Instructions:

Drain red peppers and measure 1/2 cup. In a food processor or blender, put the garlic and peppers and process until smooth. Add the Italian seasonings, olive oil, and tomato sauce. Process until blended properly. Ready to be used in recipes for pie, spaghetti, or as a substitute for tomato sauce. It can be cooled for 2 to 3 days or frozen before ready for usage.

# 285- Worcestershire Sauce

Preparation time: 5 minutes

Cooking Time: 5 minutes

Servings: 6

Difficulty Level: Easy

## Nutritional Information:

Calories: 3.9 kcal, protein: 0 g, carbohydrates: 1 g, Fat: 0 g, Cholesterol: 0 mg, Fiber: 0 g, Sodium: 40 mg, Potassium: 136 mg, Phosphorus: 10.2 mg, Calcium: 18.2 mg

## Ingredients:

- Ground black pepper to taste.
- ½ cup of apple cider vinegar
- 1 tbsp of Brown Sugar

- 2 tbsp of water
- ¼ tsp of onion powder
- 2 tbsp of soy sauce
- ¼ tsp of ground cinnamon
- 1 tsp of mustard powder
- ¼ tsp of garlic powder

## Instructions:

In a saucepan, mix the water, apple cider vinegar, soy sauce, mustard powder, brown sugar, onion powder, black pepper, garlic powder, and ground cinnamon; boil it and cook for around 45 seconds until fragrant. At room temperature, cool it.

# 286- Shallot Vinaigrette

Preparation time: 10 minutes

Cooking Time:  5 minutes

Servings: 17

Difficulty Level: Easy

## Nutritional Information:

Calories: 124  kcal, protein: 0.08 g, carbohydrates: 0.45 g, Fat: 14 g, Cholesterol: 0 mg, Fiber: 0.06 g, Sodium: 5 mg, Potassium: 10 mg, Phosphorus: 2 mg, Calcium: 4 mg

## Ingredients:

- 1 tsp of Dijon mustard
- 2/3 cup of extra virgin olive oil
- 3 tbsp of vinegar
- 1 shallot minced.
- Cracked black pepper.

## Instructions:

Mix all the ingredients in the processor, except the oil. To emulsify, slowly add oil and serve when done.

# 287- Roasted Tomatillo Salsa

Preparation time: 5 minutes

Cooking Time:  15 minutes

Servings: 6

Difficulty Level: Easy

## Nutritional Information:

Calories: 20  kcal, protein: 0 g, carbohydrates: 2 g, Fat: 1 g, Cholesterol: 0 mg, Fiber: 3 g, Sodium: 6 mg, Potassium: 86 mg, Phosphorus: 10 mg, Calcium: 4 mg

## Ingredients:

- 3 jalapenos
- 1 bunch of cilantro
- 1/4 cup of Lime juice (or to taste)
- 1 head garlic
- 1/4 cup of water or to desired consistency
- 1 lb. tomatillos (about 15-17)

## Instructions:

Halve the tomatillos. Grease the baking sheet and place jalapenos, tomatillos, and garlic on it. Gently toss the vegetables with oil. Broil the tomatillos for 10-15 minutes so that they turn brown. Take it out from the oven. In a food processor, mix all until smooth. Serve over burritos, enchiladas, or tacos, with corn chips.

# 288- French Dressing

Preparation time:5minutes

Cooking Time: 0 minutes

Servings:7

Difficulty Level: Easy

## Nutritional Information:

Calories: 73 kcal, protein:0.6g, carbohydrates:2.3 g, Fat: 6.8 g, Cholesterol: 0 mg, Fiber: 0 g, Sodium: traces, Potassium: 23 mg, Phosphorus: 4.9 mg, Calcium: 1 mg

## Ingredients:

- 4 tablespoons olive oil
- 2 tablespoons wine vinegar
- 1 tablespoon mustard
- ¼ teaspoon pepper
- 1 heaped teaspoon clear pasteurized honey
- 1 crushed clove of garlic

## Instructions:

Put all the ingredients into a small screw-top jar and shake vigorously. Keep refrigerated & shake before use.

## 289- Cornichon Pickles, Low Salt

Preparation time: 5 minutes

Cooking Time: 30 minutes

Servings: 24

Difficulty Level: Easy

## Nutritional Information:

Calories: 5 kcal, protein: 0 g, carbohydrates: 1 g, Fat: 0 g, Cholesterol: 0 mg, Fiber: 1 g, Sodium: 177 mg, Potassium: 50 mg, Phosphorus: 7 mg, Calcium: 5 mg

## Ingredients:

- 1/2 tsp of mustard seeds
- 3 cups of pickling cucumbers or cornichon
- Four sprigs of fresh tarragon
- 1 tbsp of kosher salt
- White vinegar

## Instructions:

Thoroughly wash the cucumbers and dry them. Leave the cucumbers intact if small. If they're longer than your thumb, split them lengthwise. Put and combine well with the salt in a ceramic bowl. Let it rest for 24 hours (do not refrigerate). Rinse and drain the fluids quickly, and dry cucumbers. Put into jars directly, fill three-quarters full, or place into one wide jar or crock o, leaving a gap of 2 inches between the cucumbers and the top of the bottle. The tarragon and mustard seeds are added. Cover with white vinegar at least 1-inch above the cucumbers. Cover the jars and keep them for 3-4 weeks in a cold location.

## 290- Salt-Free Sweet Brown Mustard

Preparation time:5minutes (24 hours to set)

Cooking Time: 10 minutes

Servings:1 ½ cups

Difficulty Level: Easy

## Nutritional Information:

Calories: 27 kcal, protein:0 g, carbohydrates: 4 g, Fat:1 g, Cholesterol: 0 mg, Fiber: 0 g, Sodium: 2 mg, Potassium: 27 mg, Phosphorus: 18 mg, Calcium: 9mg

## Ingredients:

- 2 teaspoons cornstarch
- 1 cup cider vinegar
- ½ cup dry mustard
- ½ cup light brown sugar
- ½ teaspoon white pepper (or black pepper)

## Instructions:

Dissolve cornstarch in a small amount of vinegar. Heat remaining vinegar; add mustard, sugar, and pepper. Stir until dissolved. When hot, add

cornstarch and cook until thick. Remove from
heat. Cover the mixture and let it stand at room
temperature for 24 hours to develop flavor.

# CHAPTER 10

## Salad Recipes

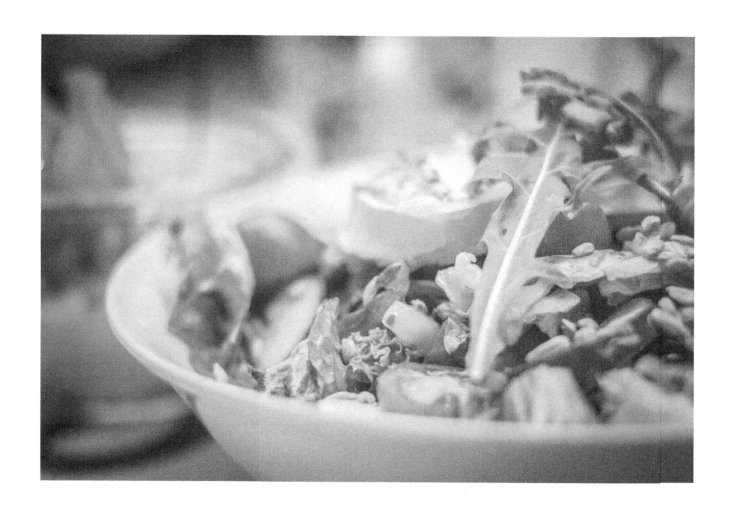

# 291- Creamy Fruit Salad

Preparation time: 45 minutes

Cooking Time: 0 minutes

Servings: 14

Difficulty Level: Easy

## Nutritional Information:

Calories: 174 kcal, protein: 2 g, carbohydrates: 19 g, Fat: 10 g, Cholesterol: 34 mg, Fiber: 2.3 g, Sodium: 40 mg, Potassium: 175 mg, Phosphorus: 43 mg, Calcium: 36 mg

## Ingredients:

- 1/2 cup of fresh berries
- 2 apples; medium size
- 1 tbsp of sour cream
- 15 ounces of canned peaches (light syrup)
- 2 fresh pears; medium
- 1-1/4 cup of heavy cream
- 1-1/2 cups of strawberries; fresh
- 4 ounces of cream cheese; low-fat
- 1-1/2 cups of green grapes
- 2 tbsp of sugar

## Instructions:

Slice peaches, pears, apples, and strawberries. Place them in a large bowl. Only put back. Put the hand mixer's metal beater and bowl in the freezer for 15 to 30 minutes. Then blend heavy cream with chilled beaters in a cooled bowl and beat until firm peak forms. Mix the sour cream, cream cheese, and sugar in a medium bowl until creamy texture forms. Then fold in the whipped cream softly. Pour the cream cheese mixture over the fruit before eating, then swirl gently. Place berries on top and serve.

# 292- Spinach-Mandarin Salad

Preparation time: 10 minutes

Cooking Time: 0 minutes

Servings: 5

Difficulty Level: Easy

## Nutritional Information:

Calories: 157 kcal, protein: 2 g, carbohydrates: 31 g, Fat: 4 g, Cholesterol: 0 mg, Fiber: 2.9 g, Sodium: 145 g, Potassium: 232 mg, Phosphorus: 32 mg, Calcium: 28 mg

## Ingredients:

- 5-ounce can of water chestnuts, drained.
- 1/4 cup of crunchy chow Mein noodles
- 1 tsp of black pepper
- 1/4 cup of vinaigrette salad dressing
- 2 cups of fresh spinach
- 1/2 cup of dried cranberries, sweetened.
- 1 apple; medium size
- 1 cup of mandarin oranges

## Instructions:

Drain the chestnuts and oranges with water and cut the apples into chunks. Put in a 1-quart serving bowl and wash drained spinach leaves. Sprinkle dried cranberries. Add the mandarin oranges, apple wedges, chow Mein noodles, and water chestnuts. Drizzle pepper. Cover and refrigerate. With 1/4-cup vinaigrette salad dressing, toss gently and eat.

# 293- Chicken Crunchy Salad

Preparation time: 2 hours 10 minutes

Cooking Time: 0 minutes

Servings: 6

Difficulty Level: Easy

## Nutritional Information:

Calories: 127 kcal, protein: 16 g, carbohydrates:2 g, Fat: 6 g, Cholesterol: 75 mg, Fiber: 0.2 g,

Sodium: 95 mg, Potassium: 136 mg, Phosphorus: 122 mg, Calcium: 14 mg

## Ingredients:

- 1 large egg; hardboiled
- 2 cups chicken, cooked.
- 1/4 tsp black pepper
- 2 tbsp onion
- 1/2 tsp sugar
- 1/4 cup of celery
- 1 tsp of fresh lemon juice
- 1/4 cup of low-fat mayonnaise.

## Instructions:

Shred or dice chicken. Slice celery, egg, and onion. In a wide bowl, put all the ingredients and mix. Before serving, cool overnight or at least for 2 hours.

## 294  Lemon Orzo Spring Salad

Preparation time:5minutes

Cooking Time: 10 minutes

Servings:4

Difficulty Level: Easy

## Nutritional Information:

Calories: 330 kcal, protein: 6 g, carbohydrates: 28 g, Fat: 22 g, Cholesterol: 3 mg, Fiber: 5 g, Sodium: 79 mg, Potassium: 376 mg, Phosphorus: 134 mg, Calcium: 67 mg

## Ingredients:

- ½ tsp of red pepper flakes
- ¼ cup of red peppers, fresh and diced.
- ½ tsp of black pepper
- ¾ cup or ¼ box of orzo pasta
- ½ cup of red or Vidalia onion; fresh and diced.
- ¼ cup of yellow peppers; fresh and diced.
- 2 cups of fresh zucchini, medium-cubed

- ½ tsp of dried oregano
- and ¼ cup of green peppers, fresh and diced.
- 3 tbsp of lemon juice; fresh
- ¼ cup and 2 tbsp of olive oil
- 1 tsp. of lemon zest
- 2 tbsp. Fresh rosemary, chopped.
- 3 tbsp of Parmesan cheese; grated.

## Instructions:

Boil orzo pasta, drain, and allow it to set. On a medium-high flame, sauté the onions, zucchini, and peppers with 2 tablespoons of oil in a wide skillet until translucent. Add 1⁄4 cup of olive oil, lemon juice, cheese, lemon zest, pepper, rosemary, red pepper flakes, and oregano to a large bowl. Then add orzo pasta and sautéed vegetables and fold them until well combined. Refrigerate it or serve.

## 295- Turkey Waldorf Salad

Preparation time: 10 minutes

Cooking Time: 0 minutes

Servings: 6

Difficulty Level: Easy

## Nutritional Information:

Calories: 200 kcal, protein:17 g, carbohydrates: 8 g, Fat: 11 g, Cholesterol: 60 mg, Fiber: 1.9 g, Sodium: 128 mg, Potassium: 296 mg, Phosphorus: 136 mg, Calcium: 26 mg

## Ingredients:

- 2 tbsp apple juice
- 12 ounces of turkey breast unsalted, cooked.
- 1 cup of celery
- 3 red apples; medium size
- 1/4 cup of mayonnaise
- 1/2 cup of onion

## Instructions:

Chop onions finely, Slash turkey into cubes, and dice apples and celery. Combine celery, turkey, onion, and apple in a medium bowl. Add apple juice and mayonnaise until well mixed and stir together. Chill before serving.

## 296- Crunchy Quinoa Salad

Preparation time:5 minutes

Cooking Time: 15 minutes

Servings: 8

Difficulty Level: Easy

## Nutritional Information:

Calories: 158 kcal, protein: 5 g, carbohydrates: 16 g, Fat: 9 g, Cholesterol: 2 mg, Fiber: 2.3 g, Sodium: 46 mg, Potassium: 237 mg, Phosphorus: 129 mg, Calcium: 61 mg

## Ingredients:

- ½ head Bibb lettuce or Boston separated and divided into cups.
- 1 cup of quinoa, rinsed.
- 5 cherry tomatoes, diced.
- 2 cups of water
- 3 green onions, chopped.
- ½ cup of cucumbers, diced and seeded.
- ½ cup of parsley, chopped.
- ¼ cup of fresh mint, chopped.
- 1 tbsp of lemon zest, grated.
- 2 tbsp of fresh lemon juice
- and ¼ cup of parmesan cheese, grated.
- 4 tbsp olive oil

## Instructions:

Wash the quinoa until clean under cool running water and drain it properly. Over medium-high heat, put the quinoa in a pan and cook for 2 minutes, stirring constantly. Pour 2 cups of water into the pan to get it to boil. Cover pans for 8-10 minutes to cook it on low heat. Fluff it

with a fork. Combine the spices, herbs, olive oil, lemon juice, and zest with the onions, tomatoes, and cucumbers. Then add the cooled quinoa to it. Pour the mixture into lettuce cups and spread parmesan cheese on top.

## 297- French Grated Carrot Salad with Lemon Dijon Vinaigrette

Preparation time: 10 minutes

Cooking Time: 0 minutes

Servings: 8

Difficulty Level: Easy

## Nutritional Information:

Calories: 61 kcal, protein: 1 g, carbohydrates: 7 g, Fat: 4 g, Cholesterol: 0 mg, Fiber: 1 g, Sodium: 88 mg, Potassium: 197 mg, Phosphorus: 22 mg, Calcium: 2 mg

## Ingredients:

- 2 tsp of Dijon mustard
- 1 scallion finely sliced.
- 9 small carrots peeled.
- 2 Tbsp extra virgin olive oil
- 1 Tbsp lemon juice
- ¼ tsp salt
- 1-2 tsp honey to taste.
- 2 Tbsp parsley, chopped.
- ¼ tsp freshly ground pepper to taste.

## Instructions:

In a food processor, grate the carrots. Mix the lemon juice, Dijon mustard, pepper, salt, olive oil, and honey in a salad dish. Add the carrots, fresh scallion, and parsley, and toss well. Cover, refrigerate, or serve it.

Note: You can add sugar, depending on the sweetness of the carrots.

# 298- Tuna Salad

Preparation time: 10 minutes

Cooking Time: 0 minutes

Servings: 4

Difficulty Level: Easy

## Nutritional Information:

Calories: 202 kcal, protein: 27 g, carbohydrates: 3 g, Fat: 9 g, Cholesterol: 36 mg, Fiber: 0.8 g, Sodium: 188 mg, Potassium: 318 mg, Phosphorus: 183 mg, Calcium: 20 mg

## Ingredients:

- 5 ounces canned low sodium, water-packed tuna
- 1/4 cup of mayonnaise
- 1/2 cucumber, medium
- 1 tbsp of fresh lime juice
- 2 fresh jalapeño peppers
- 1 tbsp fresh cilantro
- 2 green onions

## Instructions:

Cut the jalapeño peppers finely. Chop the cilantro, cucumber, and green onions. Combine the lime juice, mayonnaise, and jalapeño in a medium dish. Add drained tuna, green onions, and cucumber to it. Mix thoroughly. Refrigerate it. Serve with bread or a bagel. If needed, garnish it with chopped cilantro.

# 299- Blackberry Spinach Salad

Preparation time:5 minutes

Cooking Time: 0 minutes

Servings: 4

Difficulty Level: Easy

## Nutritional Information:

Calories: 117 kcal, protein: 4 g, carbohydrates: 5 g, Fat: 9 g, Cholesterol: 11 mg, Fiber: 2 g, Sodium: 313 mg , Potassium: 245 mg, Phosphorus: 120 mg, Calcium: 86 mg

## Ingredients:

- 1/2 cup of blackberries, fresh
- 4 cups of spinach, fresh
- 5–6 almonds toasted or raw (optional)
- 2 tbsp of cooked bacon
- 1/4 cup of balsamic vinaigrette
- 2 tbsp of feta cheese
- 2 green onion stalks

## Instructions:

Combine all the fresh ingredients and add bacon, dressings, and feta before serving.

# 300- Hawaiian Chicken Salad

Preparation time: 10 minutes

Cooking Time: 0 minutes

Servings: 4

Difficulty Level: Easy

## Nutritional Information:

Calories: 310 kcal, protein: 16.8 g, carbohydrates: 9.6 g, Fat: 23.1 g, Cholesterol: 3 mg, Fiber: 1.1 g, Sodium: 200 mg , Potassium: 260 mg, Phosphorus: 134 mg, Calcium: 10 mg

## Ingredients :

- 1-1/4 Cups of Lettuce (Shredded Head)
- 1/2 Cup of Diced Celery
- 1-1/2 Cups of Chicken (Cooked and Chopped)
- 1/2 tsp. of Sugar
- 1 Cup of Pineapple Chunks (Unsweetened and Drained)

- 1/2 cup of Mayonnaise
- 2 tsp of lemon Juice
- 1/4 tsp. of Pepper / Paprika
- Dash of Tabasco Sauce

## Instructions:

In a dish, add lettuce, celery, pineapple, and chicken. Mix lemon juice, sugar, Tabasco, pepper, and mayonnaise in a separate bowl. Add this to the mixture of chicken and toss to combine well. Serve and dust with paprika.

# 301- Strawberry Wedge Salad

Preparation time:5minutes

Cooking Time: 20 minutes

Servings: 4

Difficulty Level: Easy

## Nutritional Information:

Calories: 168 kcal, protein: 2 g, carbohydrates: 5 g, Fat: 16 g, Cholesterol: 1 mg, Fiber: 1 g, Sodium: 14 mg , Potassium: 195 mg, Phosphorus: 85 mg, Calcium: 50 mg

## Ingredients:

- 1/4 tsp of salt-free garlic powder
- 1 cup of strawberries (washed and halved)
- 3 tbsp olive oil
- 1/4 tsp of chipotle powder, salt-free
- Freshly ground black pepper
- 1/2 cup sour cream
- Head of butter lettuce leaves (washed and separated)
- Handful dill finely chopped.

## Instructions:

Preheat the oven to 375 degrees Fahrenheit. Mix the strawberries with garlic, a tablespoon of oil, and chipotle powder in a shallow bowl. Mix it

with your hand unless the strawberries are nicely coated. Then use parchment paper to cover an oven sheet and spread out the strawberry slices in a single layer. Put the mixture in the oven and bake for 12 to 15 minutes.

Add the pepper, sour cream, 1 tablespoon of water, and the remaining two tablespoons of oil to another small bowl for the dressing. To mix a milky dressing, use a fork or whisk. Add a little splash of water if it is too dense for perfect consistency. Then add the dill and give it another soft whirl until all the green bits are mixed. Serve it.

# 302- Cold Turkey Rice Salad

Preparation time: 10 minutes

Cooking Time: 20 minutes

Servings: 4

Difficulty Level: Easy

## Nutritional Information:

Calories: 288 kcal, protein:15 g, carbohydrates: 28 g, Fat: 7 g, Cholesterol: 34 mg, Fiber: 3 g, Sodium: 83 mg , Potassium: 180 mg, Phosphorus: 45 mg, Calcium: 50 mg

## Ingredients:

- 1 tbsp of olive oil
- 2 tbsp of rice vinegar
- 1 tbsp of honey
- 2 tbsp of lime juice
- 3 ½ cups of wild or brown rice, cooked.
- 1 tsp of ground ginger
- 1 ½ cups of skinless, boneless, cooked, chopped turkey breast.
- 1 bunch of green onions (½ cup) (chopped)
- 1/3 cup of dried cranberries

## Instructions:

Use turkey from a previous dinner or prepare by roasting 2 turkey cutlets in the oven. Brush it with oil and put them in a shallow pan. Cook for 15-20 minutes in preheated oven to 350 degrees F. Cool and slice into small pieces. Whisk the vinegar, oil, lime juice, ginger, and honey together in a small bowl. Combine the cooked rice, cranberries, green onion, and turkey in a side dish. Toss the ginger dressing with it and serve it.

## 303- Beet Salad

Preparation time: 10 minutes

Cooking Time: 55 minutes

Servings: 4

Difficulty Level: Easy

### Nutritional Information:

Calories: 283 kcal, protein: 6 g, carbohydrates: 16 g, Fat: 16 g, Cholesterol: 1 mg, Fiber: 3.8 g, Sodium: 241 mg , Potassium: 393 mg, Phosphorus: 102 mg, Calcium: 8.9 mg

### Ingredients:

- 2-3 ounces of Stilton or blue cheese
- 4, beets (peeled, roasted, chilled, and diced)
- 1/4 cup of fresh basil chopped fine.
- 1/2 cup of pecans or walnuts
- 1/2 cup of fruit or herb vinegar
- Lettuce leaf :1 per person
- 2 tablespoons of olive oil

### Instructions:

Heat the oven to 400°F. Bake beets until soft for 45 mins and cool, peel, and slice them. In a saucepan, add the sugar, water, and nuts. Heat the mixture, stirring continuously until most liquid bubbles are absorbed. Place nuts on aluminum foil until coated and the frying pan is dry. Let it cool, and it can be kept for many months at room temperature. Put up a lettuce bed. Toss the vinegar, basil, and oil with the beets. Spread it on a lettuce bed. Sprinkle nuts and cheese cubes over it. Serve.

## 304  Quinoa Salad with Fresh Mozzarella

Preparation time: 10 minutes

Cooking Time: 15 minutes

Servings: 8

Difficulty Level: Easy

### Nutritional Information:

Calories: 158 kcal, protein: 5 g, carbohydrates: 16 g, Fat: 9 g, Cholesterol: 2 mg, Fiber: 2.3 g, Sodium: 46 mg , Potassium: 237 mg, Phosphorus: 129 mg, Calcium: 61 mg

### Ingredients:

- ¼ cup of red onion, diced.
- 1 cup of cooked quinoa
- 1 red bell pepper, diced.
- 1 cup of cherry tomatoes, halved.
- 1 yellow pepper diced.
- 1 cup of frozen sweet peas
- 1/8 cup of fresh parsley, chopped.
- 1 small zucchini or cucumber, diced.
- fresh mozzarella (about ¾ cup)

**For the Dressing (to taste):**

- 1/8 teaspoon of fresh pepper (or 3 grinds)
- ½ lemon, squeezed.
- 2 tbsp of extra virgin olive oil
- 1 tbsp of orange juice
- ½ tsp of mustard
- 1 tsp of garlic, minced.
- ½ tsp of dried oregano
- 1 ½ tbsp of balsamic vinegar

## Instructions:

Rinse the quinoa for about 2 minutes. Add quinoa and 2 cups of water to a medium pot and boil it. Lower the heat and cover when water starts boiling. Simmer for 15. Remove from the heat without removing the lid and hold covered for some more minutes until the quinoa is soft but still chewy. Around each grain, a white spiral-like string will appear. With a fork, fluff it aside to cool in a large mixing cup.

Dice all the vegetables and combine all ingredients except cheese. Add quinoa, vegetables,1/2 of the dressing, and cheese. Until you have the taste you want, add more dressing.

## 305- Cucumber and Radish Salad

Preparation time: 30 minutes

Cooking Time: 0 minutes

Servings: 4

Difficulty Level: Easy

## Nutritional Information:

Calories: 78 kcal, protein: 6 g, carbohydrates: 9 g, Fat: 2 g, Cholesterol: 7 mg, Fiber: 3 g, Sodium: 49 mg , Potassium: 389 mg, Phosphorus: 93 mg, Calcium: 87 mg

## Ingredients:

- Two sprigs of fresh tarragon
- 1 garlic clove
- 12 large red radishes
- 1 large cucumber
- 1/2 teaspoon of ground black pepper
- 1/2 cup of light sour cream
- 1 teaspoon of white vinegar

## Instructions:

Chop the tarragon and mince the garlic. Slice the cucumber and the radishes thinly. Combine the vinegar, garlic, black pepper, and sour cream in a mixing cup. Mix the sour cream mixture with the cucumber and radishes. Before serving, marinate for 20 minutes in the refrigerator. Divide the salad into four bowls and cover with sliced tarragon.

## 306- Broccoli Salad

Preparation time: 40 minutes

Cooking Time: 0 minutes

Servings: 4

Difficulty Level: Easy

## Nutritional Information:

Calories: 104 kcal, protein: 5.9 g, carbohydrates: 7.9 g, Fat: 5.3 g, Cholesterol: 15 mg, Fiber: 1.3 g, Sodium: 278 mg , Potassium: 176 mg, Phosphorus: 50.9 mg, Calcium: 35 mg

## Ingredients:

- 1 large carrot peeled and grated.
- 4 cups of broccoli sliced.
- 4 thinly sliced scallions
- 1 1/2 cup of red cabbage sliced thinly.
- 2 Tbsp. sesame seeds
- 1/4 cup of raisins

**Dressing:**

- 2 1/2 Tbsp. lite mayonnaise
- 1 Tbsp. apple cider vinegar
- 1 Tbsp. dried basil
- Dash of cayenne pepper
- 1 tsp. garlic powder

## Instructions:

Put grated carrots, broccoli florets, sliced scallions, cabbage, sesame seeds, and raisins in a wide dish. Toss well. Combine lite mayo, apple cider vinegar, garlic powder, cayenne pepper, and basil in a small bowl or measuring cup. Stir and pour in a large bowl over the vegetables. Toss to let the vegetables be coated with dressing. To allow flavors to combine, refrigerate for 30 minutes and then toss well before serving.

# 307- Cranberry Fluff Salad

Preparation time: 10 minutes

Cooking Time: 0 minutes

Servings: 4

Difficulty Level: Easy

## Nutritional Information:

Calories: 313 kcal, protein: 4.1 g, carbohydrates: 54 g, Fat: 11 g, Cholesterol: 0 mg, Fiber: 3.1 g, Sodium:73 mg , Potassium: 212 mg, Phosphorus: 65 mg, Calcium: 16 mg

## Ingredients:

- 1/2 cup of sugar
- 12 oz. of fresh cranberries
- 2 cups of mini marshmallows
- 1 cup of heavy cream
- 8 oz. of crushed pineapple, drained.

## Instructions:

In a food processor, blend cranberries. Stir in a bowl. Combine it with sugar, cover, and refrigerate overnight. Add pineapple and marshmallows that are well-drained, and mix them. Whip heavy cream. Fold the cream into the cranberry mixture with a rubber spatula. Serve cool.

# 308- Creamy Grape Salad

Preparation time: 10 minutes

Cooking Time: 0 minutes

Servings: 4

Difficulty Level: Easy

## Nutritional Information:

Calories: 98.9 kcal, protein: 2.1 g, carbohydrates: 19.5 g, Fat: 5.2 g, Cholesterol: 9.5 mg, Fiber: 1 g, Sodium: 36 mg , Potassium: 194.2 mg, Phosphorus: 4.12 mg, Calcium: 3.36 mg

## Ingredients:

- 8 oz. cream cheese
- 6 cups. grapes
- 1/2 tsp. vanilla extract
- 8 oz. sour cream softened to room temperature.
- 1/2 cup. powdered sugar

## Instructions:

Rinse grapes and combine heavy cream, cream cheese, and vanilla extract in a large mixing bowl and then add sugar and grapes; combine until mixed uniformly. Refrigerate until they are chilled, and serve it.

# 309- Green Pea Salad

Preparation time:10 minutes

Cooking Time: 0 minutes

Servings: 4

Difficulty Level: Easy

## Nutritional Information:

Calories: 132 kcal, protein: 6 g, carbohydrates: 9 g, Fat: 8 g, Cholesterol: 116 mg, Fiber: 6 g, Sodium: 209 mg , Potassium: 120 mg, Phosphorus: 103 mg, Calcium: 54 mg

## Ingredients:

- 1 medium green bell pepper; diced.
- 2 stalks of celery; diced.
- 1 can of green peas (salt-free)
- 1 red onion or sweet onion chopped.
- 1 head iceberg lettuce; chopped.
- 4 boiled eggs, sliced.
- 3/4 cup. of mayonnaise

- 2 slices bacon or turkey bacon (Cook and crumble in pieces.)
- 1/2 cup. Of shredded cheese

## Instructions:

Cut one head of lettuce and layer it in a glass bowl. Mix diced onion, celery, green bell peppers, peas, and boiled eggs. Thoroughly coat them with mayonnaise. Cover with plastic wrap and put overnight in the refrigerator. Garnish them with bacon bits and grated cheese before eating.

## 310- Apple Salad

Preparation time: 5 minutes

Cooking Time: 0 minutes

Servings: 6

Difficulty Level: Easy

## Nutritional Information:

Calories: 246 kcal, protein: 4 g, carbohydrates: 46 g, Fat: 6 g, Cholesterol: 0 mg, Fiber: 3 g, Sodium: 73 mg , Potassium: 209 mg, Phosphorus: 96 mg, Calcium: 21 mg

## Ingredients:

- 3 Tbsp. low-fat, plain yogurt
- 1/2 cup. golden raisins
- 2 cups diced apples (about 4 apples)
- 3 Tbsp. mayonnaise
- 1/2 cup. Chopped walnuts.

## Instructions:

Cut apples into cubes and mix all ingredients. Refrigerate to serve it cool.

## 311- Cabbage Slaw

Preparation time: 10 minutes

Cooking Time: 0 minutes

Servings: 6

Difficulty Level: Easy

## Nutritional Information:

Calories: 104 kcal, protein: 1 g, carbohydrates: 9 g, Fat: 8 g, Cholesterol: 1 mg, Fiber: 3 g, Sodium: 45 mg , Potassium: 287 mg, Phosphorus: 16.9 mg, Calcium: 44 mg

## Ingredients:

- 2 Cups of Red Cabbage, shredded
- 3 Cups of Green Cabbage, shredded
- 1/2 Cup of Cilantro chopped and washed.
- 2 Cups of Carrots, shredded
- 3 Tbsp. of Olive Oil
- 4 Tbsp. of Fresh Lime Juice squeezed.

## Instructions:

Mix all the ingredients in a bowl and toss until well combined. For cabbage to get soft and flavors combined, set it aside for 1-2 hours.

# CHAPTER 11

## Soup Recipes

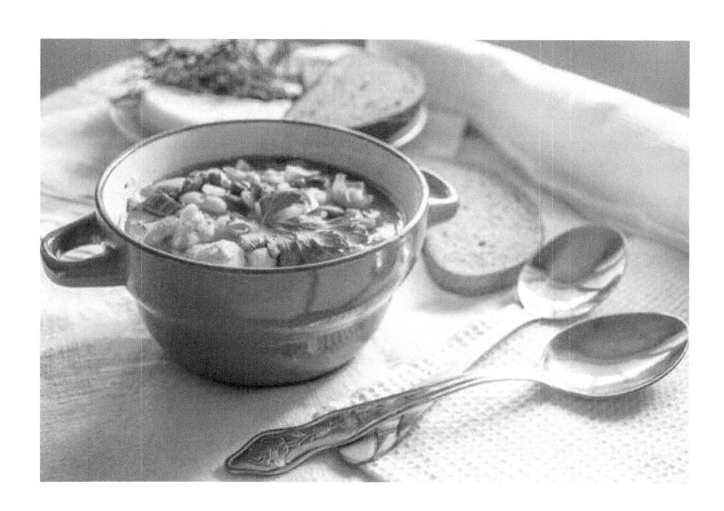

## 312- Rotisserie Chicken Noodle Soup

Preparation time: 5 minutes

Cooking Time: 30 minutes

Servings: 10

Difficulty Level: Easy

### Nutritional Information:

Calories: 186 kcal, protein: 21 g, carbohydrates: 14 g, Fat: 5 g, Cholesterol: 64 mg, Fiber: 1.5 g, Sodium: 362 mg , Potassium: 295 mg, Phosphorus: 162 mg, Calcium: 21 mg

### Ingredients:

- 3 tablespoons of fresh parsley
- 1/2 cup of onion
- 1 rotisserie chicken; cooked
- 6 ounces of wide noodles, uncooked
- 1 cup of carrots
- 8 cups of low-sodium chicken broth
- 1 cup of celery

### Instructions:

Remove bones and cut chicken into fine pieces, and measure 4 cups. In a large stockpot, pour the chicken broth and bring it to a boil. Start cutting the carrots, onion, and celery into fine pieces. To the stockpot, add vegetables, noodles, and chicken. Boil it for 15 minutes until the noodles are cooked. Serve with chopped parsley.

## 313- Salmon Soup

Preparation time: 5 minutes

Cooking Time: 30 minutes

Servings: 8

Difficulty Level: Easy

### Nutritional Information:

Calories: 155 kcal, protein: 14 g, carbohydrates: 9 g, Fat: 7 g, Cholesterol: 37 mg, Fiber: 0.5 g, Sodium: 113 mg , Potassium: 369 mg, Phosphorus: 218 mg, Calcium: 92 mg

### Ingredients:

- 1/4 cup of water
- 2 tbsp of unsalted butter
- 1/2 cup of celery
- 1 carrot; medium
- 1 pound of sockeye salmon; cooked.
- 1/2 cup of onion
- 2 cups of low-fat milk; 1%
- 2 cups of low-sodium chicken broth.
- 1/4 cup of cornstarch
- 1/8 tsp of black pepper

### Instructions:

Cut carrot, onion, and celery. In a 3-quart saucepan, melt butter over medium-high heat. Add vegetables and simmer until soft. Then add pre-cooked salmon pieces. Stir in the chicken broth, black pepper, and milk; do not boil. Low the flame to simmer. Combine the water and cornstarch. Slowly add into the broth and stir; until soup thickens. Simmer for five more minutes. Serve it hot.

## 314- Taco Soup

Preparation time: 10 minutes

Cooking Time: 7 hours

Servings: 10

Difficulty Level: Medium

### Nutritional Information:

Calories: 190 kcal, protein: 21 g, carbohydrates: 19 g, Fat: 3 g, Cholesterol: 42 mg, Fiber: 4.3 g, Sodium: 421 mg , Potassium: 444 mg, Phosphorus: 210 mg, Calcium: 28 mg

## Ingredients:

- 2 cups of low-sodium chicken broth
- 1 tbsp of Low Sodium Taco Seasoning
- 1-1/2 pounds of chicken breast boneless, skinless
- 15.25 ounces of low-sodium white corn; canned
- 15.5 ounces of dark red kidney beans; canned
- 15.5 ounces of yellow hominy; canned
- 1/2 cup of onion
- 1 cup of tomatoes(diced) with green chilies.
- 1/2 cup of green bell peppers
- 1 medium jalapeno
- 1 garlic clove

## Instructions:

Hominy, kidney beans, and corn are washed and rinsed. Chop green peppers and onions and sliced jalapeño pepper and garlic. Put the chicken in a wide crock-pot at the bottom and cover it with all the remaining ingredients. Cook for 1 hour, then reduce heat and simmer for 6 hours. Shred chicken and combine with ingredients. Pour onto the serving cup and enjoy.

## 315- Ground Beef Soup

Preparation time: 10 minutes

Cooking Time: 40 minutes

Servings: 6

Difficulty Level: Easy

## Nutritional Information:

Calories: 222 kcal, protein: 20 g, carbohydrates: 19 g, Fat: 8 g, Cholesterol: 52 mg, Fiber: 4.3 g, Sodium: 170 mg , Potassium: 448 mg, Phosphorus: 210 mg, Calcium: 43 mg

## Ingredients:

- 2 tsp of lemon pepper seasoning blend
- 1/2 cup of onion
- 1-pound of lean ground beef
- 1 cup of reduced-sodium beef broth.
- 1 tsp of browning and seasoning sauce
- 1/3 cup of white rice, uncooked
- 2 cups of water
- 1 tbsp of sour cream
- 3 cups of frozen mixed vegetables (carrots, peas, green beans, and corn)

## Instructions:

Cut onion and add with ground beef in a wide saucepan, cook until it browns, then drains fat. Add browning sauce, seasoning, broth, mixed herbs, water, and rice. Boil it on high heat and lower it to medium-low; cover and simmer for 30 minutes. Take off from heat and serve with sour cream.

## 316- Beef Barley Stew

Preparation time: 1 hour 20 minutes

Cooking Time: 2 hours 30 minutes

Servings: 6

Difficulty Level: Medium

## Nutritional Information:

Calories: 246 kcal, protein: 22 g, carbohydrates: 21 g, Fat: 8 g, Cholesterol: 51 mg, Fiber: 6.3 g, Sodium: 222 mg , Potassium: 369 mg, Phosphorus: 175 mg, Calcium: 30 mg

## Ingredients:

- 1 tsp onion herb seasoning
- 1 cup of pearl barley, uncooked
- 1 large stalk of celery
- ½ cup of onion
- 2 medium carrots
- 1 garlic clove

- 2 tbsp of all-purpose white flour
- 2 tbsp of canola oil
- ½ tsp of salt
- ¼ tsp of black pepper
- 2 bay leaves
- 1 lb. of lean beef stew meat

## Instructions:

Dip the barley for 1 hour in 2 cups of water. Cut the celery and onion. Mince a clove of garlic. Slice the carrots into wide rounds of 1/4-inch. Cube beef into 1-1/2-inch chunks. Put the stew meat, flour, and black pepper in a plastic bag. Shake it. Heat the oil in a heavy 4 L pot and cook the meat. Take the meat out of the pot and put it aside.

For 2 minutes, stir and sauté the onion, garlic, and celery in the beef drippings. And add 2L of water to get it to boil. Set the meat back in the pot, and add salt and bay leaves. Lower the heat to a boil. The barley is rinsed and drained and returned to the pot. For 1 hour, cook it and stir after every 15 mins.

Add the seasonings and sliced carrots after 1 hour. For another hour, simmer it. To avoid sticking, add additional water if required. Serve it hot.

## 317- Hungarian Sour Cherry Soup

Preparation time: 10 minutes

Cooking Time: 15 minutes

Servings: 4

Difficulty Level: Easy

## Nutritional Information:

Calories: 144 kcal, protein: 2 g, carbohydrates: 25 g, Fat: 4 g, Cholesterol: 12 mg, Fiber: 1 g, Sodium: 57 mg , Potassium: 144 mg, Phosphorus: 40 mg, Calcium: 47 mg

## Ingredients:

- 3 cups of water
- 1-1/2 cup of fresh cherries
- 1/3 cup of sugar
- 1/2 cup of low-fat sour cream.
- 1 tbsp all-purpose white flour
- 1/16 tsp salt

## Instructions:

Cut the pits from the cherries. Add the water, cherries, salt, and sugar to a medium saucepan. Boil it and then cook for 10 minutes at very low heat. For garnish, reserve 2 teaspoons of liquid and set aside. Take out more liquid of 1/4 cup and allow it to cool slightly. Then mix the sour cream and flour and add to the saucepan. Simmer over low heat for another 5 minutes. Remove from the heat and let it cool. Serve in a cup. As a garnish, stir in the reserved cherry juice.

## 318- Simple Chicken Broth

Preparation time: 10 minutes

Cooking Time:  3 hours 30 minutes

Servings: 8 cups

Difficulty Level: Easy

## Nutritional Information:

Calories: 38 kcal, protein: 5 g, carbohydrates: 3 g, Fat: 1 g, Cholesterol: 0 mg, Fiber: 1 g, Sodium: 72 mg , Potassium: 206 mg, Phosphorus: 72 mg, Calcium: 10 mg

## Ingredients:

- 2 onions, halved.
- 3 pounds whole chicken or chicken wings
- 1 celery rib, halved.
- 8 peppercorns, whole
- 2 carrots, halved.
- 2 bay leaves

- 2 tsp of dried thyme

## Instructions:

Put all ingredients with approximately 16 cups of cold water in a large pot. Boil it and simmer. Skim down the foam that gets to the top. Simmer for 3 hours. Take out chicken meat, discard other solids, and use a sieve to pour the soup. Vegetables, chicken, and grains are added. For 30 minutes, boil.

## 319- French onion soup

Preparation time: 5 minutes

Cooking Time: 50 minutes

Servings: 6

Difficulty Level: Easy

## Nutritional Information:

Calories: 76 kcal, protein: 1.9 g, carbohydrates: 4.9 g, Fat: 5.4 g; Cholesterol: 17.8 mg, Fiber: 0.1 g, Sodium: 108.1 mg , Potassium: 14 mg, Phosphorus: 33.7 mg, Calcium: 47.6 mg

## Ingredients:

- 6 cups of chopped onions.
- 2 tsp of olive oil
- 6 cups of low-sodium beef broth
- 2 tbsp of fresh thyme
- 2 ounces of gruyere cheese; shredded
- 2 cups of water
- 2 tbsp of low-sodium soy sauce
- 1/4 tsp of ground black pepper
- 2 bay leaves

## Instructions:

Heat the olive oil in a wide soup pot over medium to high heat. Add onions and sauté, stirring continuously, for 5 minutes. Turn the heat to medium and cook until caramelized for 15 to 20 minutes. Add the water, broth, bay

leaves, pepper, soy sauce, and thyme. For 20 minutes, boil. Take out bay leaves.

Preheat the oven. In 8 individual oven-proof soup pots, pour soup and cover with cheese. On a baking sheet, put the pots. Broil the soup until the cheese is melted for around 1 minute; serve it.

## 320- Black-eyed Pea Soup

Preparation time: 5 minutes

Cooking Time: 20 minutes

Servings: 6

Difficulty Level: Medium

## Nutritional Information:

Calories: 155 kcal, protein: 5 g, carbohydrates: 27 g, Fat: 3 g, Cholesterol: 0 mg, Fiber: 3 g, Sodium: 242 mg , Potassium: 318 mg, Phosphorus: 83 mg, Calcium: 35 mg

## Ingredients:

- ½ tsp of dried sage
- Two leeks, white and light green parts only, cut into ¼-inch rounds.
- 3-14-ounce cans of low-salt chicken broth.
- Two tsp of olive oil or butter
- Optional: 3 boneless chicken breasts, baked and shredded
- 1-15-ounce can of black-eyed peas, rinsed.

## Instructions:

Over medium-high, heat the oil or butter in a large pot. Add the leeks, then cook and mix until tender (about 3 minutes). Stir in the sage and cook until aromatic (for 30 seconds). Stir in the broth, fire up to high heat, cover, and bring to a simmer. Add black-eyed peas (and chicken optional) and cook until heated (approximately 3 mins). Serve it warm. Overall period is dependent on the use of pre-cooked chicken.

# 321- Curried Carrot Soup

Preparation time: 10 minutes

Cooking Time: 40 minutes

Servings: 6

Difficulty Level: Easy

## Nutritional Information:

Calories: 316 kcal, protein: 3 g, carbohydrates: 18 g, Fat: 28 g, Cholesterol: 1 mg, Fiber: 6 g, Sodium: 201 mg , Potassium: 531 mg, Phosphorus: 239 mg, Calcium: 63 mg

## Ingredients:

- 1 medium onion, diced.
- 3 tbsp of avocado oil
- 6 cups of baby carrots
- 3 cups of low sodium vegetable broth
- 1 1/2 tbsp of finely chopped fresh ginger.
- 1/2 tsp of red pepper flakes to taste.
- 1 can (15 oz) of coconut milk plus 6 tablespoons for garnish.
- 1/4 tsp of black pepper to taste.
- 1/4 tsp of sea salt to taste.
- 1 1/2 tbsp of curry powder

**Garnish:**

- 3 tbsp chives are finely chopped.
- 6 tbsp coconut cream can be whipped or drizzled on top.

## Instructions:

Add the avocado oil to a pot and heat it over medium heat. When warmed, add the diced onion, and cook for around 5-10 minutes, until soft and fragrant. Then, add minced ginger and baby carrots and simmer for 5 minutes until the ginger is aromatic.

After this, add the vegetable broth and coconut milk with the red pepper flakes and curry powder. Boil carrots for 15-20 minutes until they soften. Use an electric mixer to blend the soup to a creamy and smooth texture. Season with salt and pepper to taste. Garnish with finely chopped chives and a tablespoon of coconut cream before serving.

# 322- Mushroom Soup

Preparation time: 5 minutes

Cooking Time: 20 minutes

Servings: 6

Difficulty Level: Easy

## Nutritional Information:

Calories: 127 kcal, protein: 3 g, carbohydrates: 13 g, Fat: 8 g, Cholesterol: 0 mg, Fiber: 2 g, Sodium: 109 mg , Potassium: 299 mg, Phosphorus: 71 mg, Calcium: 56 mg

## Ingredients:

- 1/4 cup of minced onion
- 3 Tbsp of unsalted butter
- 1/4 cup of mushrooms minced.
- 1/2 cup of low sodium chicken broth.
- 1/2 cup of almond milk (unsweetened)
- Pepper to taste
- 2 1/2 Tbsp of flour (all-purpose)
- sea salt

## Instructions:

Heat butter over medium heat in a 10-inch pan. Then onion is added and sautéed until tender. Add the mushrooms, mix, and simmer for around five minutes. Sprinkle the flour on top of the vegetables and simmer for two minutes. Whisk in the milk and broth and swirl until smooth. Boil it and cook for around 5 minutes until thick.

## 323- Corn and Fennel Soup

Preparation time: 5 minutes

Cooking Time: 30 minutes

Servings: 12

Difficulty Level: Easy

### Nutritional Information:

Calories: 112 kcal, protein: 3 g, carbohydrates: 22 g, Fat: 3 g, Cholesterol: 4 mg, Fiber: 2.6 g, Sodium: 16 mg , Potassium: 298 mg, Phosphorus: 76 mg, Calcium: 20 mg

### Ingredients:

- 2 tbsp vegetable oil
- shrimp shells
- 1 kg frozen corn
- 1 celery chopped stalk.
- 2 chopped onions/leeks.
- 6 cloves garlic
- black pepper to taste.
- 2 cups chopped fennel.
- 2 liters of cold water
- tarragon to taste

### Instructions:

In oil, sauté shrimp shells until they turn pink. Add the celery, onion, garlic, corn, and fennel, and continue cooking until the onions are translucent and the flavor starts to form. Stir in liquid and get it to a simmer, and let it boil for 30 minutes at least. To extract unnecessary fibers, process soup in a mixer and strain. Garnish with fresh tarragon and ground black pepper.

## 324- Vegetable and Lentil Soup

Preparation time: 10 minutes

Cooking Time: 25 minutes

Servings: 4

Difficulty Level: Easy

### Nutritional Information:

Calories: 190 kcal, protein: 11 g, carbohydrates: 25 g, Fat: 6 g, Cholesterol: 3 mg, Fiber: 7 g, Sodium: 198 mg , Potassium: 468 mg, Phosphorus: 139 mg, Calcium: 53 mg

### Ingredients:

- ½ sweet onion, diced.
- 1 tbsp of extra-virgin olive oil
- Juice of 1 lemon
- 2 carrots, diced.
- ½ cup lentils
- 2 celery stalks, diced.
- 5 cups of low-sodium chicken broth or chicken stock
- Black pepper, freshly ground, to taste.
- 2 cups of chard leaves, sliced.

### Instructions

Heat olive oil in a wide stockpot over medium-high heat. Add onion and whisk until tender, 3 to 5 minutes. Add the celery, carrots, lentils, and broth. Boil it, lower the heat, and cook until the lentils are soft and uncovered for 15 minutes. Add the chard and cook until wilted, for an additional 3 minutes. Add the lemon juice and pepper and serve it.

## 325- Cauliflower and Pear Soup

Preparation time: 10 minutes

Cooking Time: 40 minutes

Servings: 8

Difficulty Level: Easy

### Nutritional Information:

Calories: 192 kcal, protein: 2.5 g, carbohydrates: 35.9 g, Fat: 5.8 g, Cholesterol: 4 mg, Fiber: 5 g, Sodium: 192.6 mg , Potassium: 375.6 mg, Phosphorus: 51.7 mg, Calcium: 16 mg

## Ingredients:

- 2 Pear, Bartlett (peeled and diced).
- 1 (750g) Cauliflower (1 whole head of cauliflower)
- 3 Apples, golden peeled and diced.
- 3 Tbsp of Olive oil
- ¼ cup of Honey
- 1Onions, chopped.
- 2 Tbsp of Cider Vinegar
- 1Tbsp of Garlic
- 6 cups of Vegetable stock
- 1 Carrot, chopped.
- 2 tsp of Cloves, ground
- 2 Tbsp of Ginger, fresh, peeled and chopped.
- 6 sprigs Thyme, fresh
- 8 pieces of Croutons for garnish

## Instructions:

Slice the cauliflower and medium-sized pieces of carrots and onions. Peel the pears and apples and cut them into large chunks. Add the oil to the pan and sweat the pears and vegetables for 10-15 minutes. Add the ginger, cloves, vegetable stock, and cider vinegar. Boil and cook for fifteen minutes. Add mixture and thyme to the processor, then add water or more vegetable stock to change the texture. As a garnish and for a good crunch, add croutons.

## 326- Traditional Chicken-Vegetable Soup

Preparation time: 20 minutes

Cooking Time: 35 minutes

Servings: 6

Difficulty Level: Easy

## Nutritional Information:

Calories: 124 kcal, protein: 15 g, carbohydrates: 4 g, Fat: 5 g, Cholesterol: 46 mg, Fiber: 1 g, Sodium: 92 mg , Potassium: 231 mg, Phosphorus: 132 mg, Calcium: 24 mg

## Ingredients:

- ½ sweet onion, diced.
- 1 tablespoon of unsalted butter
- 2 teaspoons of minced garlic
- 1 carrot, diced.
- 2 celery stalks, chopped.
- 1 cup of Chicken Stock
- 4 cups of water
- Freshly ground black pepper
- 2 tablespoons of chopped fresh parsley.
- 1 teaspoon of chopped fresh thyme.

## Instructions:

In a large pot over medium heat, melt the butter. Sauté the onion and garlic until softened, about 3 minutes. Add the celery, carrot, chicken, chicken stock, and water. Bring the soup to a boil, reduce the heat, and simmer for about 30 minutes or until the vegetables are tender. Add the thyme; simmer the soup for 2 minutes. Season with pepper and serve topped with parsley.

## 327- Spring Vegetable Soup

Preparation time:5minutes

Cooking Time: 1 hour 10 minutes

Servings:2

Difficulty Level: Easy

## Nutritional Information:

Calories: 114 kcal, protein: 2g, carbohydrates:13 g, Fat: 6g, Cholesterol: 0 mg, Fiber: 3.4 g, Sodium: 262 mg, Potassium: 400 mg, Phosphorus: 108mg, Calcium: 48 mg

## Ingredients:

- 1 cup fresh green beans
- 3/4 cup celery
- 1/2 cup onion
- 1/2 cup carrots

- 1/2 cup mushrooms
- 1/2 cup frozen corn
- 1 medium Roma tomato
- 2 tablespoons olive oil
- 4 cups low-sodium vegetable broth
- 1 teaspoon dried oregano leaves
- 1 teaspoon garlic powder
- 1/4 teaspoon salt

## Instructions:

Remove tips and strings from the green beans and cut them into 2-inch pieces. Dice the celery, onion, carrots, mushrooms, and tomato. Heat the olive oil and sauté the celery and onion in a large pot until tender. Add the remaining ingredients and bring to a boil. Reduce heat to a simmer and cook for 45 to 60 minutes.

## 328- Turkey-Bulgur Soup

Preparation time: 25 minutes

Cooking Time: 45 minutes

Servings: 6

Difficulty Level: Easy

## Nutritional Information:

Calories: 124 kcal, protein: 11 g, carbohydrates: 8 g, Fat:5 g, Cholesterol: 41 mg, Fiber: 2 g, Sodium: 89 mg , Potassium: 207 mg, Phosphorus: 102 mg, Calcium: 27 mg

## Ingredients:

- ½ sweet onion, chopped.
- ½ pound cooked ground turkey, 93% lean
- 1 teaspoon of olive oil
- 4 cups of water
- 1 teaspoon of garlic minced.
- 1 celery stalk, chopped.
- 1 cup of Easy Chicken Stock (here)
- ½ cup of bulgur
- 1 carrot sliced thin.
- ½ cup shredded green cabbage.

- 2 dried bay leaves
- 1 teaspoon of chopped fresh sage.
- 2 tablespoons of chopped fresh parsley.
- 1 teaspoon of chopped fresh thyme.
- Freshly ground black pepper
- Pinch red pepper flakes

## Instructions:

Place a large saucepan over medium-high heat and add the olive oil. Sauté the turkey for about 5 minutes or until the meat is cooked. Add the onion, garlic, and sauté for about 3 minutes or until the vegetables are softened. Add the bulgur, chicken stock, water, carrot, celery, cabbage, and bay leaves. Boil it, reduce the heat to low, and cook for about 35 minutes or until the vegetables and bulgur are tender. Take out the bay leaves and stir in the sage, parsley, red pepper flakes, and thyme. Use pepper to season it and serve it.

## 329- Cream of Chicken with Wild Rice Asparagus Soup

Preparation time: 10 minutes

Cooking Time: 55 minutes

Servings: 2 cups

Difficulty Level: Easy

## Nutritional Information:

Calories: 295 kcal, protein: 21 g, carbohydrates: 28 g, Fat: 11 g, Cholesterol: 45 mg, Fiber: 3.3 g, Sodium: 385 mg, Potassium: 527 mg, Phosphorus: 252 mg, Calcium: 183 mg

## Ingredients:

- 3/4 cup of long-grain & wild rice blend
- 2 cups of asparagus
- 1 cup carrots
- 1/2 cup onion

- 4 cups of almond milk; unsweetened & unenriched
- 3 garlic cloves
- 1/4 cup unsalted butter
- 1/2 teaspoon of salt
- 4 cups of chicken broth; low-sodium
- 1/2 teaspoon of thyme
- 1/2 teaspoon of fresh ground pepper
- 1/4 teaspoon of nutmeg
- 1 bay leaf
- 1/2 cup of all-purpose flour
- 1/2 cup of vermouth; extra dry
- 2 cups of cooked chicken

## Instructions:

Prepare the long grain and wild rice blend according to package instructions, omitting salt and seasoning packet if included. After removing the pan from the heat, leave the rice to set for 15 minutes. Cool off and set aside.

Cut the onion, carrots, and asparagus into dice. Chop up the garlic. In a Dutch oven, melt the butter and cook garlic and onion until they are soft. Add spices, herbs, and carrots. Over medium heat, continue to cook until soft. Mix flour and cook over low heat for 10 mins. Pour in four cups of chicken broth & vermouth. Using a wire whisk, blend until smooth.

Dice the cooked chicken into small pieces. Add chicken and asparagus to the soup, then slowly add the almond milk. Simmer for 20 minutes. Fold in prepared rice and serve.

## 330- Minestrone Soup

Preparation time: 15 minutes

Cooking Time: 30 minutes

Servings: 1 cup

Difficulty Level: Easy

## Nutritional Information:

Calories: 144 kcal, protein: 5.9 g, carbohydrates: 21.9 g, Fat: 4.3 g, Cholesterol: 1 mg, Fiber: 2.8 g, Sodium: 55.1 mg, Potassium: 355.2 mg, Phosphorus: 97.8 mg, Calcium: 51.3 mg

## Ingredients:

- 1½ cup of Macaroni; elbow-shaped, dry
- 14-ounce Tomatoes, diced; No Salt Added
- 4 cups of Chicken Broth, Low Sodium, Low Fat
- 2 large celery stalks
- 1 tsp of leaves Oregano - Dried
- 2 cloves Garlic
- 1 tsp of ground Black Pepper
- ½ large Onion
- 1 tsp of leaves Basil; Dried
- ½ cup of chopped Zucchini
- 1 large Carrot
- 1 can of Green Snap Beans; no salt added
- 2 tablespoons of Olive Oil

## Instructions:

Slice up zucchini, onion, and garlic. Slice the carrot. Clean canned green beans or use 1 1/2 cups of freshly cut beans. Warm the olive oil in a wide pot or Dutch oven on medium heat. For 2-3 minutes, cook onions until transparent. Add the zucchini, carrot, celery, and garlic. (If using fresh beans, add green beans.) Cook the vegetables for about 5 minutes, or until they soften. Add oregano, black pepper, basil, and canned green beans. Add chicken broth and one can of diced, salt-free tomatoes. Simmer after bringing to a boil. Cook for ten minutes. Add and cook pasta for 8 to 10 minutes as directed on the packet. Add a fresh basil sprig as a garnish. Enjoy after spooning it into a bowl!

## 331- Cream of Crab Soup

Preparation time: 5 minutes

Cooking Time: 20-30 minutes

Servings: 1 cup

Difficulty Level: Easy

## Nutritional Information:

Calories: 130 kcal, protein: 12 g, carbohydrates: 7 g, Fat: 6 g, Cholesterol: 53 mg, Fiber: 0.4 g, Sodium: 212 mg, Potassium: 312 mg, Phosphorus: 80 mg, Calcium: 86 mg

## Ingredients

- 1 tablespoon unsalted butter
- 1 medium onion
- 1/2-pound fresh lump crab meat
- 4 cups low-sodium chicken broth
- 1 cup half & half creamer
- 2 tablespoons cornstarch
- 1/4 teaspoon Old Bay Seasoning
- 1/8 teaspoon dill weed
- 1/8 teaspoon black pepper

## Instructions:

In a wide pot over medium heat, melt the butter. Add chopped onion to the pot. Stirring occasionally, cook onion until tender and translucent, then add crab meat. Cook for 2 to 3 minutes, stirring constantly. Add chicken broth and bring the mixture to a boil. Reduce heat to low. Combine half & half creamer and cornstarch in a small bowl. Whisk until smooth. Add to soup, turn up the heat, and stir until the mixture thickens and boils. Pepper, Old Bay spice, and dill weed are added to the soup. Serve it warm

## 332- Thai Pumpkin Soup

Preparation time: 5 minutes

Cooking Time: 30 minutes

Servings: 7

Difficulty Level: Easy

## Nutritional Information:

Calories: 139 kcal, protein: 4 g, carbohydrates: 14 g, Fat: 9 g, Cholesterol: 0 mg, Fiber: 3 g, Sodium: 168 mg, Potassium: 368 mg, Phosphorus: 75 mg, Calcium: 37 mg

## Ingredients:

- 1 onion minced
- 1 clove garlic minced
- 2 Tbsp. brown sugar
- 1/4 tsp of black pepper
- 2 cups of vegetable broth; low sodium
- 1 tsp curry powder
- 1/2 tsp coriander
- 1/4 tsp of salt
- 1/2 tsp ground cinnamon
- 1 15oz can of coconut milk; low fat (lite)
- 1/8 tsp ground nutmeg
- 1 15oz can of pumpkin puree
- 1/4 tsp powdered ginger
- 1/4 cup creamy peanut butter
- 1/2 cup fresh cilantro chopped

## Instructions:

In a large saucepan, cook garlic, onion, and brown sugar in olive oil until soft. Add salt, broth, and pepper. Boil it. Reduce the heat to low and cook until onions get soft, occasionally stirring, for about 15 mins. Add coconut milk, peanut butter, pumpkin, and remaining spices. Cook them until warm, 5 mins. Transfer the soup to a blender to blend until smooth, or use an immersion blender. Serve with cilantro garnished on top.

# CHAPTER 12

## Drinks and Smoothies

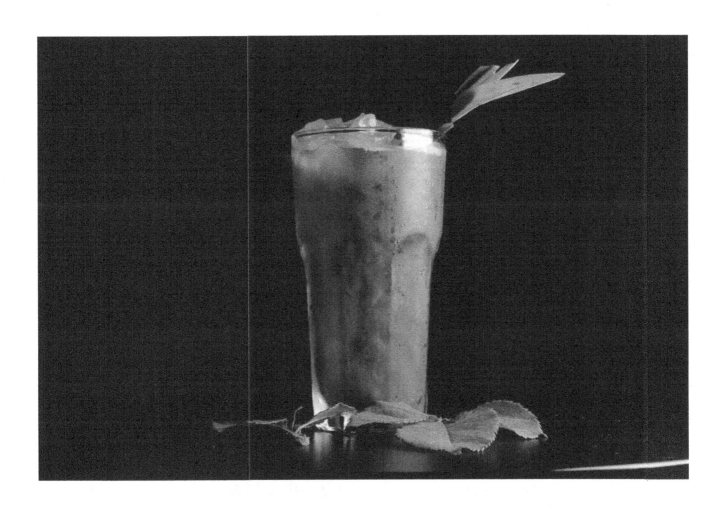

## 333- Blackberry-Sage Flavored Water

Preparation time: 5 minutes

Cooking Time: 0 minutes

Servings: 10

Difficulty Level: Easy

### Nutritional Information:

Calories: 7 kcal, protein: 0 g, carbohydrates: 2 g, Fat: 0 g, Cholesterol: 0 mg, Fiber: 0.7 g, Sodium: 7 mg, Potassium: 26 mg, Phosphorus: 3 mg, Calcium: 13 mg

### Ingredients:

- 4 sage leaves
- 1 cup of blackberries: fresh
- 10 cups of water

### Instructions:

Smash blackberries. Use a pitcher to incorporate all the ingredients. Before serving, refrigerator overnight.

## 334 Beet and Apple Juice Blend

Preparation time: 5 minutes

Cooking Time: 0 minutes

Servings: 2

Difficulty Level: Easy

### Nutritional Information:

Calories: 53 kcal, protein: 1 g, carbohydrates: 13 g, Fat: 0 g, Cholesterol: 0 mg, Fiber: 0 g, Sodium: 66 mg, Potassium: 338 mg, Phosphorus: 36 mg, Calcium: 36 mg

### Ingredients:

- 1/4 cup of parsley
- 1 medium fresh carrot: medium
- 1/2 apple: medium
- 1 celery stalk
- 1/2 beet: medium

### Instructions:

In a juicer, put the beet, apple, celery, parsley, and carrot; process them for juice extraction. Drink it fresh or put it to cool in the refrigerator.

## 335- Citrus Shake

Preparation time: 5 minutes

Cooking Time: 0 minutes

Servings: 2

Difficulty Level: Easy

### Nutritional Information:

Calories: 190 kcal, protein: 7 g, carbohydrates: 36 g, Fat: 2 g, Cholesterol: 1.5 mg, Fiber: 1.3 g, Sodium: 194 mg, Potassium: 312 mg, Phosphorus: 85 mg, Calcium: 204 mg

### Ingredients:

- 1 cup of orange sherbet
- 1/2 cup of pineapple juice
- 1/2 cup of egg product: low-cholesterol
- 1/2 cup of almond milk: unsweetened

### Instructions:

In a processor, add all the ingredients and process them for 30 seconds. Enjoy fresh or freeze to use later.

## 336- Rice Milk

Preparation time: 10 minutes

Cooking Time: 0 minutes

Servings: 4

Difficulty Level: Easy

## Nutritional Information:

Calories: 84 kcal, protein: 1 g, carbohydrates: 20 g, Fat: 0 g, Cholesterol: 0 mg, Fiber: 0.2 g, Sodium: 1 mg, Potassium: 22 mg, Phosphorus: 26 mg, Calcium: 6 mg

## Ingredients:

- 3 cups of filtered water.
- 1-1/2 cup of cooked rice
- 1 tsp of vanilla extract
- 2 tbsp of sugar

## Instructions:

Add the filtered water, cooked rice, sugar, and vanilla to a blender. Blend for 4 minutes at high speed or until the mixture is milky and the rice is mixed thoroughly. Strain the mixture with a cheesecloth. And dump the solid rice. Add rice milk into a pot, cover, and refrigerate. Before serving, shake the pot.

## 337- Cucumber-Lemon Flavored Water

Preparation time: 10 minutes

Cooking Time: 0 minutes

Servings: 7

Difficulty Level: Easy

## Nutritional Information:

Calories: 4 kcal, protein: 0 g, carbohydrates: 1 g, Fat: 0 g, Cholesterol: 0 mg, Fiber: 0.4 g, Sodium: 7 mg, Potassium: 37 mg, Phosphorus: 5 mg, Calcium: 16 mg

## Ingredients:

- 10 cups of water
- 1 cucumber: medium
- 1/4 cup of fresh mint leaves
- 1 lemon
- 1/4 cup of fresh basil leaves

## Instructions:

Cut the cucumber and lemon thinly. Chop the mint leaves and basil finely. Use a pitcher to incorporate all the ingredients. Before you serve it, refrigerate it overnight.

## 338- Hot Cocoa

Preparation time: 10 minutes

Cooking Time: 0 minutes

Servings: 1

Difficulty Level: Easy

## Nutritional Information:

Calories: 72 kcal, protein: 1 g, carbohydrates: 13 g, Fat: 3 g, Cholesterol: 0 mg, Fiber: 1.8 g, Sodium: 10 mg, Potassium: 100 mg, Phosphorus: 49 mg, Calcium: 26 mg

## Ingredients:

- 3 tbsp of whipped cream
- 1 cup hot water
- 2 tsp of sugar: granulated
- 1 tbsp cocoa powder: unsweetened
- 2 tbsp of cold water

## Instructions:

Mix the sugar and cocoa powder in a cup. To make a thin paste, add cold water and blend. Then add a cup of hot water to dissolve the paste. Garnish with whipped cream.

## 339- Hot Apple Cider

Preparation time: 5 minutes

Cooking Time: 0 minutes

Servings: 16

Difficulty Level: Easy

## Nutritional Information:

Calories: 44 kcal, protein: 0 g, carbohydrates: 11 g, Fat: 0 g, Cholesterol: 0 mg, Fiber: 0.1 g, Sodium: 22 mg, Potassium: 88 mg, Phosphorus: 6 mg, Calcium: 8 mg

## Ingredients:

- 6 whole cloves
- 4 cups of apple juice
- 1/2 tsp of allspice
- 1 cinnamon-flavored tea bag
- 4 cups of cranberry juice: low-sugar
- 1 tsp of pumpkin pie spice
- 2 cinnamon sticks

## Instructions :

In a Crock-Pot, add all the ingredients. Let it be steep for an hour or more, and take out a teabag. Serve it.

## 340- Green Juice

Preparation time: 5 minutes

Cooking Time: 0 minutes

Servings: 2

Difficulty Level: Easy

## Nutritional Information:

Calories: 130 kcal, protein: 1 g, carbohydrates: 31 g, Fat: 1 g, Cholesterol: 0 mg, Fiber: 0 g, Sodium: 5 mg, Potassium: 365 mg, Phosphorus: 47 mg, Calcium: 34 mg

## Ingredients:

- 1 cucumber: medium
- 1/2 lemon
- 2 green apples: medium
- 1/2 cup of fresh pineapple

## Instructions:

Clean well all ingredients and cut apple and cucumber into cubes. Extract juice using a juicer and drink fresh.

## 341- Pineapple-Mint Flavored Water

Preparation time: 5 minutes

Cooking Time: 0 minutes

Servings: 7

Difficulty Level: Easy

## Nutritional Information:

Calories: 8 kcal, protein: 0 g, carbohydrates: 2 g, Fat: 0 g, Cholesterol: 0 mg, Fiber: 0.2 g, Sodium: 6 mg, Potassium: 22 mg, Phosphorus: 2 mg, Calcium: 8 mg

## Ingredients:

- 10 cups of water
- 12 fresh mint leaves
- 1 cup of fresh pineapple

## Instructions:

Slice pineapple and chop mint.
Use a pitcher to incorporate all the ingredients. Serve cool.

## 342- Pineapple Squash

Preparation time: 10 minutes

Cooking Time: 6-7 hours

Servings: 5

Difficulty Level: Easy

## Nutritional Information:

Calories: 80 kcal, protein: 0 g, carbohydrates: 21 g, Fat: 0 g, Cholesterol: 0 mg, Fiber: 0.1 g,

Sodium: 0 mg, Potassium: 34 mg, Phosphorus: 2 mg, Calcium: 3 mg

## Ingredients:

- 8 ounces crushed pineapple: unsweetened
- 1 tbsp butter: small pieces.
- summer squash: 1 pound
- 1/2 cup of green bell pepper
- zucchini squash: 1 pound
- 1/3 cup of brown sugar.
- 1-1/2 tsp of ground cinnamon

## Instructions:

Dice the green bell pepper and cut the squash and zucchini into 1-inch cubes. Put only squash in a 4-quart slow cooker. In a shallow bowl, combine the green bell pepper, pineapple, butter, cinnamon, and brown sugar. Then add them to the squash and mix properly and cover it. Cook for6-7 hours or until the squash is tender at low heat. Swirl gently and serve it.

## 343- Minted Lemonade

Preparation time: 5 minutes

Cooking Time: 0 minutes

Servings: 5

Difficulty Level: Easy

## Nutritional Information:

Calories: 80 kcal, protein: 0 g, carbohydrates: 21 g, Fat: 0 g, Cholesterol: 0 mg, Fiber: 0.1 g, Sodium: 0 mg, Potassium: 34 mg, Phosphorus: 2 mg, Calcium: 3 mg

## Ingredients:

- 3-1/2 cups of cold water
- 1/2 cup of sugar
- 6 tbsp of fresh lemon juice
- 6 mint leaves

## Instructions:

Mix the mint leaves, lemon juice, and sugar in a 1-quart pitcher. To fill the pitcher, add 3-1/2 cups of cool water. Until cold, freeze it. Serve with a sprig of mint in a 6-ounce bottle.

## 344 Apple-Cinnamon Flavored Water

Preparation time: 10 minutes

Cooking Time: 0 minutes

Servings: 10

Difficulty Level: Easy

## Nutritional Information:

Calories: 16 kcal, protein: 0 g, carbohydrates: 4 g, Fat: 0 g, Cholesterol: 0 mg, Fiber: 0 g, Sodium: 7 mg, Potassium: 24 mg, Phosphorus: 2 mg, Calcium: 13 mg

## Ingredients:

- 2 tsp of ground cinnamon
- 10 cups of water
- 2 cinnamon sticks
- 1 medium apple

## Instructions:

Slice the apple into small pieces without peeling. Use a pitcher to add all the ingredients. Before serving, refrigerator overnight.

## 345- Molasses Milk

Preparation time: 5 minutes

Cooking Time: 5 minutes

Servings: 1

Difficulty Level: Easy

## Nutritional Information:

Calories: 200 kcal, protein: 1 g, carbohydrates: 30 g, Fat: 9 g, Cholesterol: 1 mg, Fiber: 1 g, Sodium: 97 mg, Potassium: 211 mg, Phosphorus: 85 mg, Calcium: 304 mg

## Ingredients:

- 1/2 tbsp of blackstrap molasses
- 1 cup of rice milk: unsweetened
- dash of ground cinnamon
- 1/2 tbsp coconut oil

## Instructions:

In a saucepan, combine all the ingredients and put them on the burner over medium-low heat to heat the milk while being cautious not to make the mixture boil over. Pour the mixture into a food processor and blend for 10-15 seconds for frothy milk. For iced molasses milk, pour into a mug and drink warm or add some ice cubes.

## 346- Raspberry Pear Sorbet

Preparation time: 4 hours 15 minutes

Cooking Time: 5 minutes

Servings: 6

Difficulty Level: Easy

## Nutritional Information:

Calories: 135 kcal, protein: 0.9 g, carbohydrates: 32 g, Fat: 4 g, Cholesterol: 0 mg, Fiber: 5 g, Sodium: 3 mg, Potassium: 168 mg, Phosphorus: 27 mg, Calcium: 7 mg

## Ingredients:

- 2 large pears canned in juice: halves.
- 1-pint raspberries: fresh
- 1/2 cup of sugar
- 1/3 cup of lime juice
- Fresh raspberries (optional)

- 1 tbsp pear liqueur (optional)

## Instructions:

For a basic syrup, add 1 cup of water and sugar in a small saucepan and, boil it, stir to dissolve the sugar. Simmer for 3 minutes, uncovered. Remove from heat. Put it in the fridge to cool. Meanwhile, pear, 1-pint raspberries, pear liqueur, and lime juice are mixed in the food processor for puree. Cover; process until smooth, or for 30 seconds. Stir in chilled syrup.

Prepare or distribute the mixture in an 8x8x2-inch baking pan using ice-cream maker instructions. Cover; freeze until firm, or for 4 hours. Place the mixture in the food processor. Cover; process until smooth, or 30 seconds. Transfer the sorbet to a 1-quart freezer container; cover and freeze for 6 to 8 hours or until firm. Let it stand 5 minutes before scooping at room temperature. Serve with raspberries also. Allows a serving of 6 (1/2 cup).

## 347- Peachy Strawberry Slush Drink

Preparation time: 10 minutes

Cooking Time: 0 minutes

Servings: 3

Difficulty Level: Easy

## Nutritional Information:

Calories: 26.1 kcal, protein: 0.3 g, carbohydrates: 7 g, Fat: 0.1 g, Cholesterol: 0 mg, Fiber: 1.6 g, Sodium: 3.5 mg, Potassium: 110.3 mg, Phosphorus: 25 mg, Calcium: 6 mg

## Ingredients:

- 1 ½ cups of crushed ice.
- 4 medium peaches, pitted, peeled, and sliced.
- 1 ½ cups of plain seltzer water, chilled
- 1 tbsp of lemon juice or lime juice
- Orange peel curls (optional)

- 5-8 fresh strawberries

## Instructions:

Mix the strawberries, peaches, lemon or lime juice, and crushed ice in a blender. Cover and blend for smoothing texture. Pour the mixture of fruit into large, chilled glasses. Garnish drinks by putting fresh strawberry slices on wood dowels if desired; wrap around skewers with orange peel curls. Put skewers in your drinks.

## 348- Refreshing Cucumber and Lemon Water

Preparation time: 10 minutes

Cooking Time: 0 minutes

Servings: 10

Difficulty Level: Easy

### Nutritional Information:

Calories: 10 kcal, protein: 0.12 g, carbohydrates: 2.25 g, Fat: 0 g, Cholesterol: 0 mg, Fiber: 0.38 g, Sodium: 1.12 mg, Potassium: 0 mg, Phosphorus: 0 mg, Calcium: 5.25 mg

### Ingredients:

- 8 cups of water
- ¼ cup of basil leaves
- 1 cucumber
- ¼ cup of mint leaves
- 1 lemon

### Instructions:

Cut lemon and cucumber into thin slices and chop mint and basil leaves. To a pitcher, add all the ingredients. Cool it in the refrigerator and enjoy it.

## 349- Fresh Blueberry Lemon Smoothie

Preparation time: 5 minutes

Cooking Time: 0 minutes

Servings: 4

Difficulty Level: Easy

### Nutritional Information:

Calories: 205 kcal, protein: 2.5 g, carbohydrates: 48.9 g, Fat: 2.9 g, Cholesterol: 0 mg, Fiber: 7.8 g, Sodium: 83 mg, Potassium: 638 mg, Phosphorus: 275 mg, Calcium: 239 mg

### Ingredients:

- ½ cup of blueberries: frozen
- 1 banana: frozen
- ½ cup of strawberries or mango: frozen
- ½ lemon, squeezed.
- ½ cup of plain yogurt or milk

### Instructions:

In a food processor, blend all the ingredients. Add ice cubes, and at high speed, blend them to get a smooth texture. Serve it.

## 350- Watermelon-Rosemary Flavored Water

Preparation time: 5 minutes

Cooking Time: 0 minutes

Servings: 10

Difficulty Level: Easy

### Nutritional Information:

Calories: 4 kcal, protein: 0 g, carbohydrates: 1 g, Fat: 0 g, Cholesterol: 0 mg, Fiber: 0 g, Sodium: 7 mg, Potassium: 21 mg, Phosphorus: 2 mg, Calcium: 9 mg

### Ingredients:

- 10 cups of water
- 2 stems of fresh rosemary

- 1 cup of watermelon

## Instructions:

Slash watermelon into fine cubes. In a pitcher, add all ingredients and mix them. Before serving, cool it in the refrigerator.

# 351- Banana-Apple Smoothie

Preparation time: 5 minutes

Cooking Time: 0 minutes

Servings: 2

Difficulty Level: Easy

## Nutritional Information:

Calories: 292 kcal, protein: 9 g, carbohydrates: 61 g, Fat: 5 g, Cholesterol: 0 mg, Fiber: 5 g, Sodium: 103 mg, Potassium: 609 mg, Phosphorus: 140 mg, Calcium: 35 mg

## Ingredients:

- 2 tbsp of oat bran
- 1/2 banana peeled: chunks.
- 1/4 cup of skim milk
- 1/2 cup of plain yogurt
- 1 tbsp honey
- 1/2 cup applesauce: unsweetened

## Instructions:

Add yogurt, banana, applesauce, honey, and milk to a blender and blend to smooth texture. Then add oat bran and keep blending until thickened.

# 352- Parsley Cilantro drink

Preparation time: 5 minutes

Cooking Time: 0 minutes

Servings: 2

Difficulty Level: Easy

## Nutritional Information:

Calories: 23 kcal, protein: 2.5 g, carbohydrates: 4 g, Fat: 0.6 g, Cholesterol: 0 mg, Fiber: 3 g, Sodium: 46 mg, Potassium: 521 mg, Phosphorus: 25 mg, Calcium: 47 mg

## Ingredients:

- 1 small lemon or lime
- 1/2 cup of parsley chopped.
- 1-inch ginger root: peeled.
- 1/4 tsp of cinnamon: ground (optional)
- 1/2 cup of cilantro: chopped.
- 1 medium apple

## Instructions:

Through the juicer, pass all ingredients to extract the juice and drink it fresh. If required, add cinnamon for flavoring.

# 353- Fresh Fruit Lassi

Preparation time: 5 minutes

Cooking Time: 0 minutes

Servings: 2

Difficulty Level: Easy

## Nutritional Information:

Calories: 169 kcal, protein: 9 g, carbohydrates: 29 g, Fat: 4 g, Cholesterol: 0 mg, Fiber: 2 g, Sodium: 143 mg, Potassium: 98 mg, Phosphorus: 59 mg, Calcium: 15 mg

## Ingredients:

- 1/2 cup of milk
- 1 cup of plain yogurt
- 1/2 cup of mango juice (or peach or apricot nectar)
- 1/4 tsp of Cardamom (optional)
- 1-3 tbsp of sugar to taste.
- 1/4 cup of lime juice (optional)

## Instructions:

Add all the ingredients into the blending jar and blend it for about 2 minutes to get a smooth and thick texture. Serve it cool.

## 354  Strawberry Sorbet

Preparation time: 5 minutes

Cooking Time: 0 minutes

Servings: 4

Difficulty Level: Easy

## Nutritional Information:

Calories: 22 kcal, protein: 0 g, carbohydrates: 5 g, Fat: 0 g, Cholesterol: 0 mg, Fiber: 1.5 g, Sodium: 2 mg, Potassium: 123 mg, Phosphorus: 18 mg, Calcium: 12 mg

## Ingredients:

- 1 tbsp of lemon juice
- ¼ cup of sugar
- 1 ¼ cups of crushed or cubed ice.
- ¼ cup of water
- 1 cup of frozen or fresh strawberries, cleaned,

## Instructions:

Blend all the ingredients for sorbet in a blender until it forms a smooth texture.

## 355- Ginger Tea

Preparation time: 5 minutes

Cooking Time: 5 minutes

Servings: 2

Difficulty Level: Easy

## Nutritional Information:

Calories: 16 kcal, protein: 0.2 g, carbohydrates: 3.7 g, Fat: 0.1 g, Cholesterol: 0 mg, Fiber: 0.3 g, Sodium: 0.4 mg, Potassium: 41.8 mg, Phosphorus: 1.6 mg, Calcium: 10.6 mg

## Ingredients:

- 1 cup of water
- 1-inch chunk of fresh ginger
- Optional flavorings (choose just one):
  - 1" piece of fresh turmeric),
  - several sprigs of fresh mint
  - 1 cinnamon stick,
  - 1 teaspoon honey or maple syrup to taste.
  - 1 thin round of fresh lemon or orange,

## Instructions:

In a saucepan over a high flame, add water and ginger slices. Then add fresh mint or fresh turmeric and cinnamon stick. Boil it and lower the heat for a gentle boil for 5 minutes. Take the pot away from the heat. Carefully strain the mixture into a heat-safe liquid measuring cup or directly into a mug via a mesh sieve. Serve with a lemon ring or a drizzle of honey or maple syrup. Serve it warm.

## 356- Mixed Berry Protein Smoothie

Preparation time: 8 minutes

Cooking Time: 0 minutes

Servings: 2

Difficulty Level: Easy

## Nutritional Information:

Calories: 152 kcal, protein: 14 g, carbohydrates: 15 g, Fat: 4 g, Cholesterol: 50 mg, Fiber: 2.4 g, Sodium: 84 mg, Potassium: 216 mg, Phosphorus: 76 mg, Calcium: 79 mg

## Ingredients:

- 1 cup of frozen or fresh mixed berries
- 4 ounces of cold water
- whey protein powder: 2 scoops
- 1/2 cup of whipped cream topping.
- 2 ice cubes
- One tsp of liquid flavor enhancer: any berry flavor.

## Instructions:

Put water, frozen fruit, liquid flavor enhancer drops, and ice cubes in a blender. Blend until well mixed and slushy. Add powder protein and whipped topping and blend thoroughly. Divide into 2 servings and serve one directly, or to enjoy later, freeze and defrost.

## 357- Blueberry-Pineapple Smoothie

Preparation time: 5 minutes

Cooking Time: 0 minutes

Servings: 3

Difficulty Level: Easy

## Nutritional Information:

Calories: 155.4 kcal, protein: 7.4 g, carbohydrates: 31.1 g, Fat: 0.75 g, Cholesterol: 0 mg, Fiber: 3 g, Sodium: 104.1 mg, Potassium: 289.4 mg, Phosphorus: 27.5 mg, Calcium: 3 mg

## Ingredients:

- ½ cup of pineapple chunks
- 1 cup of blueberries: frozen
- ½ cup of cucumber
- ½ cup of water
- ½ apple

## Instructions:

Add pineapple, cucumber, water, apple, and blueberries, to a blending jar and blend to a smooth and thick texture. Serve it cool.

## 358- Bahama Breeze Smoothie

Preparation time: 5 minutes

Cooking Time: 0 minutes

Servings: 2

Difficulty Level: Easy

## Nutritional Information:

Calories: 180 kcal, protein: 2 g, carbohydrates: 44 g, Fat: 0 g, Cholesterol: 0 mg, Fiber: 2 g, Sodium: 20 mg, Potassium: 33.1 mg, Phosphorus: 2.9 mg, Calcium: 40 mg

## Ingredients:

- 1 small orange, peeled.
- ½ cup of strawberries
- handful of spinach
- ½ cup of rice milk
- ½ cup of pineapple

## Instructions:

Add orange, spinach, rice milk, pineapple, and strawberries, to a blending jar and blend to a smooth texture. Serve it cool.

## 359- Apple-Chai Smoothie

Preparation time: 40 minutes

Cooking Time: 10 minutes

Servings: 1-2

Difficulty Level: Easy

## Nutritional Information:

Calories: 129 kcal, protein: 5 g, carbohydrates: 20 g, Fat: 3 g, Cholesterol: 0 mg, Fiber: 2 g, Sodium: 133 mg, Potassium: 305.5 mg, Phosphorus: 5 mg, Calcium: 30 mg

## Ingredients:

- 2 cups of ice
- 1 cup of rice milk: unsweetened
- 1 apple, peeled, chopped.
- 1 chai tea bag

## Instructions:

Heat the rice milk in a medium saucepan for around 5 minutes over low heat. Shift the milk from heat and add the teabag. Refrigerate with the tea bag, and let the milk cool for around 30 minutes. Remove the teabag, then gently press it to release all the taste. Put the milk, apple, and ice in a blender and blend until smooth. Serve it.

## 360- Fruity Smoothie

Preparation time: 5 minutes

Cooking Time: 0 minutes

Servings: 2

Difficulty Level: Easy

## Nutritional Information:

Calories: 186 kcal, protein: 23 g, carbohydrates: 19 g, Fat: 2 g, Cholesterol: 41 mg, Fiber: 1.1 g, Sodium: 62 mg, Potassium: 282 mg, Phosphorus: 118 mg, Calcium: 160 mg

## Ingredients:

- 1 cup of crushed ice
- 8 ounces of fruit cocktail canned with juice.
- 1 cup of cold water
- 2 scoops of whey protein powder: vanilla-flavored

## Instructions:

Add ingredients to a blending jar and blend to a smooth texture. Serve it cool.

## 361- Kidney Cleanser Juice

Preparation time: 10 minutes

Cooking Time: 0 minutes

Servings: 3

Difficulty Level: Easy

## Nutritional Information:

Calories: 130 kcal, protein: 4 g, carbohydrates: 31 g, Fat: 1 g, Cholesterol: 0 mg, Fiber: 3 g, Sodium: 5 mg, Potassium: 365 mg, Phosphorus: 45 mg, Calcium: 32 mg

## Ingredients:

- 4 cups of filtered water, divided.
- 1 cup of organic cranberries
- 4 dates
- Juice of 2 organic lemons
- 2 red organic apples, sliced.
- 1 sprig of fresh organic mint or peppermint (optional)
- 1 Tbsp. of Cardamom (optional)

## Instructions:

Combine the 3 cups of water and cranberries in a medium-sized pot and boil it. Switch off the heat and allow it to cool. Mix the dates or date paste in a food processor with lemon juice and one cup of water left. Move the sliced apples and all the cranberries and water to a large glass container or jar. Stir and add the cardamom and mint leaves.

## 362- Golden milk

Preparation time: 5 minutes

Cooking Time: 5 minutes

Servings: 1

Difficulty Level: Easy

## Nutritional Information:

Calories: 291 kcal, protein: 1 g, carbohydrates: 37 g, Fat: 16 g, Cholesterol: 1 mg, Fiber: 1 g, Sodium: 96 mg, Potassium: 147 mg, Phosphorus: 75 mg, Calcium: 313 mg

## Ingredients:

- 1/4 tsp of ground cinnamon
- 1 cup almond milk: unsweetened
- 1/2 tsp of turmeric
- 1 tbsp of honey or maple syrup
- 1/8 tsp of ground black pepper
- 2 tbsp of coconut oil
- 1/4 tsp of ground ginger

## Instructions:

Combine all the ingredients in a saucepan and place it over low heat. Cook for a few minutes to infuse flavor. Enjoy warm.

## 363- Spicy Pina Colada Smoothie

Preparation time: 5 minutes

Cooking Time: 0 minutes

Servings: 2

Difficulty Level: Easy

## Nutritional Information:

Calories: 189 kcal, protein: 13.4 g, carbohydrates: 32 g, Fat: 5 g, Cholesterol: 0 mg, Fiber: 3 g, Sodium: 5 mg, Potassium: 349 mg, Phosphorus: 121 mg, Calcium: 16 mg

## Ingredients:

- ½ cup of pineapple juice, unsweetened
- 1 cup of pineapple, canned or fresh
- 1 tsp of Stevia or other sweeteners
- One pinch of red pepper flakes
- 1 cup (8 oz) of tofu, firm

## Instructions:

Add ingredients to a blending jar and blend to a smooth texture. Serve it cool.

# CHAPTER 13

## Sweets and Desserts

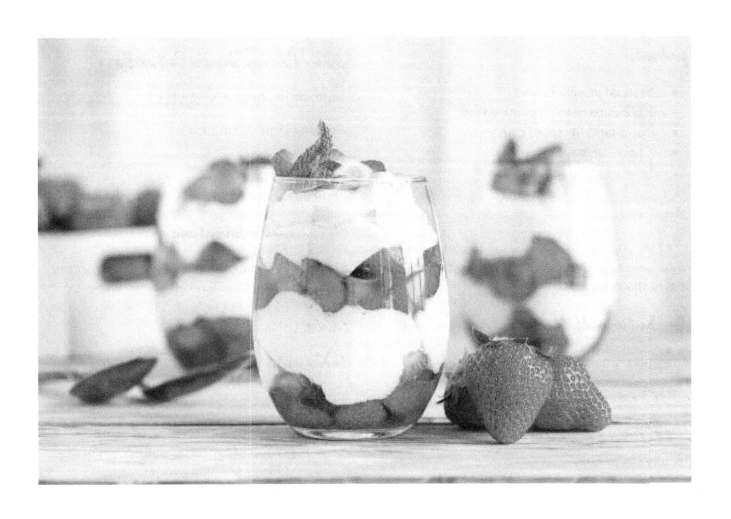

# 364- Chia Pudding

Preparation time: 4 hours 10 minutes

Cooking Time: 0 minutes

Servings: 4

Difficulty Level: Easy

## Nutritional Information:

Calories: 184 kcal, protein: 7 g, carbohydrates: 14 g, Fat: 9 g, Cholesterol: 1 mg, Fiber: 8 g, Sodium: 94 mg, Potassium: 199 mg, Phosphorus: 200 mg, Calcium: 314 mg

## Ingredients:

- 1 tsp. of vanilla extract
- 1 1/2 cups of milk: plant-based
- Optional: 1/4 tsp. of cinnamon
- 2 Tbsp. of maple syrup
- 1/2 cup of chia seeds

## Instructions:

Add all the ingredients to a mason jar. Stir well to mix. Cover and put overnight or for at least 4 hours in the refrigerator.

# 365- Buttermilk biscuits

Preparation time: 10 minutes

Cooking Time: 15 minutes

Servings: 4

Difficulty Level: Easy

## Nutritional Information:

Calories: 150 kcal, protein: 3 g, carbohydrates: 20 g, Fat: 6 g, Cholesterol: 2 mg, Fiber: 0.6 g, Sodium: 176 mg, Potassium: 56 mg, Phosphorus: 40 mg, Calcium: 30 mg

## Ingredients:

- 4 tbsp of unsalted butter
- 1 1/2 cups of plain flour (all-purpose)
- 1 tsp of baking soda
- 2 tsp of sugar
- 1/2 cup of buttermilk

## Instructions:

Mix the dried ingredients. Slice the butter until it is pea-sized. To bring the dough together, add the buttermilk. Roll out the dough and slice it into cookies. Bake for around 10 minutes at 350 ° F, or until golden.

# 366- Cherry Brown Butter Bars

Preparation time: 10 minutes

Cooking Time: 50 minutes

Servings: 16

Difficulty Level: Medium

## Nutritional Information:

Calories: 349 kcal, protein: 4 g, carbohydrates: 37 g, Fat: 21 g, Cholesterol: 84 mg, Fiber: 1 g, Sodium: 51 mg, Potassium: 116 mg, Phosphorus: 75 mg, Calcium: 18 mg

## Ingredients:

**Crust**

- 2/3 cup of sugar
- 3/4 cup of butter, unsalted and melted.
- 1/2 tsp of vanilla extract
- 1/8 tsp of salt
- 2 cups plus 2 Tbsp of flour

**Creamy Top and Cherry Filling**

- 3 eggs
- 1 cup of unsalted butter
- 2/3 cup of sugar
- 1/2 cup of flour

- 1/8 tsp of salt
- 1 tsp of vanilla extract
- 4 cups of cherries (pitted and coated with 2 tsp of flour)
- 1 tsp of almond extract

## Instructions:

Preheat the oven to 375 °F and use parchment paper to cover a 13 x 9-inch baking dish. Mix the sugar, vanilla, and melted butter in a medium bowl with a spatula. Add salt and flour, then whisk until combined. Uniformly press the dough onto the bottom of the prepared baking bowl. Bake for 18 minutes until the crust is golden and puffy. Switch to a wire rack and cool it.

Cook the butter in a large saucepan over medium heat to make the filling, stirring continuously until it foams, clears, and then becomes deep brown; it will take 6 minutes. To cool slightly, pour browned butter into a glass measuring cup. Whisk together the sugar, eggs, and salt in a medium dish. Add extracts and flour and whisk until smooth. Gradually whisk in the browned butter; whisk until thoroughly combined.

Arrange the cherries over the cooled crust and carefully spread the filling over the fruit. Bake until the filling is puffed and golden, for around 30 minutes, and a toothpick inserted in the middle comes out clean. Remove it from the pan and put them on a cutting board; use a serrated knife to cut it into squares once cooled. Store the bars in an airtight jar at room temperature for up to one day, and store any leftover bars in the freezer.

## 367- Vegan Bounty Bars

Preparation time: 45 minutes

Cooking Time: 5 minutes

Servings: 12

Difficulty Level: Medium

## Nutritional Information:

Calories: 190 kcal, protein: 2 g, carbohydrates: 10 g, Fat: 17 g, Cholesterol: 1 mg, Fiber: 3 g, Sodium: 14 mg, Potassium: 139 mg, Phosphorus: 45 mg, Calcium: 30 mg

## Ingredients:

- 1/4 cup of melted coconut oil or coconut butter (slightly warmed)
- 2 cups of shredded coconut: unsweetened
- 2 tbsp of honey or maple syrup.
- Salt to taste.
- 1/2 cup of melted chocolate chips; vegan.

## Instructions:

Add melted coconut oil or butter, shredded coconut, honey, or maple syrup, and mix until a sticky mixture forms in a food processor. Do not over-process the coconut, or it will make the bars look sandy. You can also mix it by hand with a spatula in a bowl. In a 5 X 7" or 8 X 4" loaf pan lined with parchment paper, press the coconut mixture firmly and place in the freezer until entirely stiff, for about 1 hour.

Split it into 12 bars. If the bars begin to fall apart, press them back together and freeze again before cutting; it will take another hour. Melt the chocolate over a small pot of simmering water in a microwave or a heat-proof bowl.

Dip the bars one by one into the chocolate and place them on a wire rack or pan lined with baking paper. Sprinkle sea salt on top. Allow for at least 30 minutes to set up in the refrigerator. Serve cool or refrigerate in an airtight container for up to 7 days.

## 368- Dark Chocolate Pecan Granola

Preparation time: 5 minutes

Cooking Time: 35 minutes

Servings: 8

Difficulty Level: Medium

## Nutritional Information:

Calories: 253 kcal, protein: 6 g, carbohydrates: 24 g, Fat:16 g, Cholesterol: 1 mg, Fiber: 6 g, Sodium: 79 mg, Potassium: 236 mg, Phosphorus: 105 mg, Calcium: 50 mg

## Ingredients:

- 2 tbsp of coconut oil
- 1 ¾ oz of dark chocolate (1/4 cup)
- 2 tbsp of maple syrup
- ½ cup of flax seeds: ground
- 2 cups of rolled oats.
- ¼ tsp of sea salt
- ½ cup of pecans (toasted and grated).

## Instructions:

Set the oven to 325 °F and use parchment paper to cover a baking sheet. Heat the coconut oil, maple syrup, and dark chocolate in a heat-proof bowl using a microwave. After every 30 seconds, swirl the chocolate mixture until it is fully melted. Be careful: the bowl is getting warm.

Then add the flax seeds, oats, sea salt, and pecans to the melted mixture of chocolate. To mix, whisk thoroughly. On the covered baking dish, layer the granola and bake for 20-25 minutes, flipping halfway through. As it cools, it will begin to crisp up.

## 369- Peanut Butter Maple Cookies

Preparation time: 20 minutes

Cooking Time: 20 minutes

Servings: 10

Difficulty Level: Medium

## Nutritional Information:

Calories: 112 kcal, protein: 3 g, carbohydrates: 11 g, Fat: 7 g, Cholesterol: 3 mg, Fiber: 1 g, Sodium: 57 mg, Potassium: 96 mg, Phosphorus: 25 mg, Calcium: 11 mg

## Ingredients:

- 2 tbsp of banana: mashed (about ¼ to ⅓ banana)
- ½ cup of peanut butter unsalted
- 2 tbsp of maple syrup
- 1 tsp of vanilla extract
- 2 tbsp of sugar: granulated
- ¼ cup of flour; all-purpose.
- salt to taste
- ½ tsp of baking soda

## Instructions:

Preheat an oven to 350°F and use parchment paper to cover the baking sheet. Put the peanut butter, mashed banana, sugar, maple syrup, and vanilla extract in a mixing bowl. Mix with a wooden spoon until well combined. This mixture would be dense. Mix the flour, baking soda, and salt in a separate dish. Combine wet ingredients with the dry mixture in the bowl. Blend until no flour streaks remain, and are sure not to overmix it.

Shape cookies and line them on a baking sheet into 1-tbsp balls. For flattening, use the back of a fork and create a crisscross pattern. Put in the oven and bake until the cookies have risen and the surface appears dry; it will take 12-15 minutes. Take it out from the oven and allow it to cool (about 10-15 minutes). As they cool, they'll firm up. Store in an airtight container for up to 3 days at room temperature or up to 10 days in the fridge.

## 370- Lemon Loaf

Preparation time: 10 minutes

Cooking Time: 60 minutes

Servings: 8

Difficulty Level: Easy

## Nutritional Information:

Calories: 398 kcal, protein: 5 g, carbohydrates: 54 g, Fat: 18 g, Cholesterol: 30 mg, Fiber: 0.6 g, Sodium: 129 mg, Potassium: 77 mg, Phosphorus: 70 mg, Calcium: 30 mg

## Ingredients:

- 2 tbsp of lemon zest
- 1 cup of all-purpose flour
- 4 eggs
- ½ tsp of baking soda
- ½ cup of Splenda
- 6 tbsp of lemon juice
- ½ cup of white sugar
- 1 tsp of vanilla
- ½ cup olive oil (extra virgin)

## Instructions:

Preheat the oven to 350 degrees F. Mix dry ingredients and add the lemon zest. Whisk the sugar, eggs, olive oil, vanilla, Splenda, and lemon juice in a separate dish. Through the egg mixture, fold the dry ingredients. Pour the batter into a 4x8" non-stick loaf pans and bake for around one hour.

## 371- Coconut Chocolate Almond Mousse

Preparation time: 40 minutes

Cooking Time: 0 minutes

Servings: 4

Difficulty Level: Medium

## Nutritional Information:

Calories: 292 kcal, protein: 5 g, carbohydrates: 10 g, Fat: 29 g, Cholesterol: 1 mg, Fiber: 5 g, Sodium: 17 mg, Potassium: 404 mg, Phosphorus: 52 mg, Calcium: 50 mg

## Ingredients:

- ¼ cup of cocoa powder: unsweetened
- 1 can of (13.5 oz) coconut milk; full-fat, refrigerated overnight.
- Sea salt to taste.
- 2–3 tbsp of sugar or monk fruit sweetener; powdered.
- ½ tsp of vanilla extract
- 2–3 tbsp of almond butter unsalted

**Optional toppings:** sliced almonds, grated chocolate, raspberries, or whipped coconut milk

## Instructions:

For at least 6 hours or overnight, refrigerate canned coconut milk with a whisk and mixing bowl. The fat-rich coconut cream separates and rises from the surface while the liquid portion settles down. The cream would be used for the mousse. Take the mixing bowl and coconut milk and whisk from the fridge until cooled. To hold the layers apart, open the can of coconut milk without shaking it too hard. The thick coconut cream that bubbles to the surface is scooped out and moved into the cooled bowl. Reserve remaining coconut water. To your standing or hand mixer, attach the cooled whisk and whip the coconut cream or whisk it by hand. The whipped coconut cream will start to maintain its form and curve downward but will not drip. For soft peaks, it would take about 2-3 minutes.

Add a tablespoon of coconut water from the can one at a time and whisk to get soft peaks if the coconut cream is too firm or lumpy. Sift and whip powdered sugar and cocoa powder. Add vanilla, almond butter, and sea salt. Whip to get a chocolate taste. Divide the mixture into four little cups. Cover and refrigerate. If required, add complementary toppings before serving.

## 372- Warm Apple Pie Oatmeal

Preparation time: 10 minutes

Cooking Time: 5 minutes

Servings: 6

Difficulty Level: Easy

## Nutritional Information:

Calories: 297 kcal, protein: 3 g, carbohydrates: 42 g, Fat: 13 g, Cholesterol: 32 mg, Fiber: 2.4 g, Sodium: 9.5 mg, Potassium: 193 mg, Phosphorus: 74 mg, Calcium: 35 mg

## Ingredients:

- ½ cup of rolled oats.
- 1/3 cup of milk
- 1 dash of nutmeg ground
- ½ small, diced apple,
- 1 tsp of brown sugar
- Optional: 2 tbsp of granola to garnish
- Shredded coconut
- 1 dash of cinnamon: grounded

## Instructions:

Add the oats, milk, diced apple, nutmeg, and cinnamon to a large bowl. Microwave for 1 1/2 minutes, on high. Stir. Before serving, add some brown sugar. This gives a better taste. Add shredded coconut or granola for a little crunch. Enjoy

## 373- Apple & Cherry Chutney

Preparation time: 5 minutes

Cooking Time: 30 minutes

Servings: 32

Difficulty Level: Medium

## Nutritional Information:

Calories: 55 kcal, protein: <1 g, carbohydrates: 14 g, Fat: 4 g, Cholesterol: 0 mg, Fiber: 5 g, Sodium: 2 mg, Potassium: 12 mg, Phosphorus: 1 mg, Calcium: 10 mg

## Ingredients:

- 1 cup of tart cherries; dried
- 1 tart apple; medium
- 1 red onion small, thinly sliced.
- 1 1/2 cups of sugar
- 1 cup of apple cider vinegar

## Instructions:

Core and quarter apples and cut them into thin slices without peeling them. Put apples and cherries in a large saucepan with vinegar, onions, and sugar. Cook and whisk until sugar has melted and the mixture starts to simmer.

Reduce heat to low, cover it and simmer for 8-10 minutes until the onions get soft and the dried cherries are tender and plump. Uncover and raise the heat and boil until the syrup is reduced to a glossy glaze, for around 5 more minutes. Chutney can be consumed at once, stored for many days, /refrigerate.

## 374 Peach and Yogurt Parfait

Preparation time: 5 minutes

Cooking Time: 0 minutes

Servings: 1-2

Difficulty Level: Easy

## Nutritional Information:

Calories: 260 kcal, protein: 6 g, carbohydrates: 47 g, Fat: 5 g, Cholesterol: 5 mg, Fiber: 2 g, Sodium: 170 mg, Potassium: 280 mg, Phosphorus: 120 mg, Calcium: 100 mg

## Ingredients:

- 1 cup of peach, chopped.
- 1 cup of plain yogurt: fat-free
- dashes of cinnamon
- 3 tbsp of granola

## Instructions:

Mix all ingredients and pour them into a glass. Refrigerate it and serve cool.

## 375- Sweet Custard

Preparation time: 10 minutes

Cooking Time: 20 minutes

Servings: 4

Difficulty Level: Easy

### Nutritional Information:

Calories: 123 kcal, protein: 8 g, carbohydrates: 9 g, Fat: 7 g, Cholesterol: 30 mg, Fiber: 2 g, Sodium: 98 mg, Potassium: 161 mg, Phosphorus: 157 mg, Calcium: 151 mg

### Ingredients:

- 4 eggs
- 1 cup of milk
- 1/2 tsp of vanilla extract
- 2 tbsp of sugar

### Instructions:

Preheat the oven to 325°F. Beat all ingredients together until thoroughly combined. Pour into 4 custard cups that are lightly greased. In a baking pan, position the custard cups and fill the pan with sufficiently hot water to cover the half sides of the custard cups. Custards are done when a knife comes out dry and is inserted near the middle (1 hour). Let it stand before serving for 5 minutes. Put bowls in the microwave for 7 minutes, cook at low power for 7 minutes, and turn cups when required for even cooking.

## 376- Vanilla Ice Cream

Preparation time: 15 minutes

Cooking Time: 3 minutes

Servings: 8

Difficulty Level: Medium

### Nutritional Information:

Calories: 159 kcal, protein: 3 g, carbohydrates: 22 g, Fat: 6 g, Cholesterol: 0 mg, Fiber: 0 g, Sodium: 64 mg, Potassium: 87 mg, Phosphorus: 36 mg, Calcium: 15 mg

### Ingredients:

- 1/2 cup of sugar
- 1 tbsp of vanilla extract
- 1 cup of egg product; low cholesterol
- rock salt and ice (for ice cream maker)
- 2 cups of non-dairy liquid creamer

### Instructions:

Beat the egg and sugar until well combined, utilizing a 1-quart microwaveable dish. Stir in non-dairy creamer and microwave for 1 minute, or until mixture thickens. Withdraw from the heat. Stir in the vanilla when cooled. Pour the combination into the ice cream machine's central tub. Place the rock salt and ice around the container. Process according to the manufacturer's instructions.

## 377- Lemon Curd

Preparation time: 5 minutes

Cooking Time: 15 minutes

Servings: 5

Difficulty Level: Easy

### Nutritional Information:

Calories: 99 kcal, protein: 1 g, carbohydrates: 12 g, Fat: 3 g, Cholesterol: 1 mg, Fiber: 3 g, Sodium: 9 mg, Potassium: 15 mg, Phosphorus: 13 mg, Calcium: 37 mg

## Ingredients:

- 2 cups of sugar: granulated
- 2/3 cup of lemon juice (4 lemons)
- zest from 4 lemons
- 4 whole eggs plus 1 egg yolk, beaten.
- 1 cup of butter unsalted

## Instructions:

Heat the lemon juice, zest, and sugar in a saucepan until the sugar has dissolved. Take it off from heat and add butter. When the mixture is at room temperature, gently dribble in the eggs and whisk them. Over a double boiler heat, place the mixture. When the mixture thickens, or if the internal temperature exceeds 170 degrees F, remove it. Stir the curd for 5 minutes or until thickened. A spoon can thickly coat the mixture. Pass through a good filter. Hold it in the refrigerator for around one month or use it.

## 378- Cinnamon Rice Pudding

Preparation time: 10 minutes

Cooking Time: 60 minutes

Servings: 4

Difficulty Level: Easy

## Nutritional Information:

Calories: 218 kcal, protein: 7 g, carbohydrates: 23 g, Fat: 12 g, Cholesterol: 21 mg, Fiber: 1 g, Sodium: 67 mg, Potassium: 238 mg, Phosphorus: 139 mg, Calcium: 193 mg

## Ingredients:

- 300 ml of whole milk
- 75 g of (3 oz) sugar
- 100 g of (4 oz) pearl rice or pudding rice
- 1 tsp of vanilla extract
- 300 ml of double cream
- 1 tsp of ground cinnamon
- 300 ml of water

## Instructions:

Put all the ingredients in a pan and stir well, except for the cinnamon and vanilla essence. Heat for about 1 hour on a medium to low heat setting. Stir regularly to confirm that the rice does not stick to the bottom of the pan. Stir in the vanilla essence until the rice is cooked, and add cinnamon to taste; heat for around 10 minutes, and it's done.

## 379- Almond Pecan Caramel Corn

Preparation time: 10 minutes

Cooking Time: 1 hour 10 minutes

Servings: 10

Difficulty Level: Medium

## Nutritional Information:

Calories: 595 kcal, protein: 9 g, carbohydrates: 55 g, Fat: 9 g, Cholesterol: 0 mg, Fiber: 4 g, Sodium: 150 mg, Potassium: 257 mg, Phosphorus: 144 mg, Calcium: 20 mg

## Ingredients:

- 2 cups of almonds: unblanched
- 1 cup of butter: unsalted
- 20 cups of popped popcorn or 3/4 cup of popcorn kernels
- 1/2 cup of corn syrup
- 1 cup of pecan halves
- 1 cup of granulated sugar
- 1 tsp of baking soda
- pinch of cream of tartar

## Instructions:

Popcorn is baked evenly with pecans and almonds in a broad roasting pan. Stir together the butter, sugar, tartar cream, and corn syrup in a wide thick saucepan. Bring to a boil over medium-high flame, and continuously stir it. Let it simmer without stirring for 5 minutes. Take it off from the heat and stir in the baking soda. Pour the caramel generously over the popcorn mixture, swirling until well coated. Bake for 1 hour at 200 degrees F; stir after 10 minutes. Let it cool; occasionally stir it. Store for up to one week in an airtight tin.

# 380- Chocolate Mint Cake

Preparation time: 40 minutes

Cooking Time: 50 minutes

Servings: 12

Difficulty Level: Medium

## Nutritional Information:

Calories: 354 kcal, protein: 5 g, carbohydrates: 44 g, Fat: 10 g, Cholesterol: 5 mg, Fiber: 5 g, Sodium: 231mg, Potassium: 94 mg, Phosphorus: 82 mg, Calcium: 30 mg

## Ingredients:

- 2 cups flour (all-purpose)
- 4 ounces chocolate; unsweetened
- 1 cup of water
- 1 tsp baking powder, low sodium
- 2 cups sugar
- 2 eggs
- tsp of baking soda
- 1 tsp of apple cider vinegar
- 2 tsp peppermint extract
- stick of butter: unsalted.
- 1 cup of whipping cream
- For the frosting, 1 1/2 cups of sour cream
- For the frosting, 1 1/2 cups semisweet chocolate chip

## Instructions:

Preheat the oven to 375°F. Melt the butter, chocolate, and sugar with water over medium heat in a wide saucepan. Stir periodically until the components are blended fully. Shift mixture to a wide bowl and let cool. Add the baking soda, flour, and baking powder to a medium dish. Mix the cream and apple cider vinegar in a small bowl and put it aside. When cooling the chocolate mixture, brush butter and flour on two 9-inch diameter butter cake pans. It is recommended to layer a parchment paper lining since the cake is very moist and will adhere to the pan. To the melting chocolate, add the cream and vinegar combination. Lightly combine it and substitute the eggs. Gently blend in the dry products, taking caution not to over-mix. Add the mint extract and whisk gently after all the ingredients are well combined. In baking dishes, add cake batter. Bake for 30-35 minutes on the middle rack or until the toothpick inserted into the center comes clean. Before removing it from the baking sheet, let the cake cool for up to 30 minutes. Make the frosting when the cake is cooling. Melt the chocolate chips in a double boiler until soft. Slowly add the sour cream until well combined after making the chocolate cool for a few minutes; once the cake is thoroughly cooled, frost and enjoy.

# 381- Apple caramel

Preparation time: 35 minutes

Cooking Time: 0 minutes

Servings: 6

Difficulty Level: Easy

## Nutritional Information:

Calories: 244 kcal, protein: 6 g, carbohydrates: 28 g, Fat: 12 g, Cholesterol: 2 mg, Fiber: 2.6 g, Sodium: 60 mg, Potassium: 147 mg, Phosphorus: 63 mg, Calcium: 40 mg

## Ingredients:

- 8 ounces of crushed pineapple, canned packed in juice
- 3 cups of Granny Smith apples
- 8 ounces of topping; whipped.
- 1/4 cup of butterscotch baking chips

- Unsalted peanut
- 1/2 cup of butterscotch dessert topping.

## Instructions:

Clean the apples, do not peel them. Cut apples into cubes of around 1". Thaw the whipped topping. Mix diced apples with smashed pineapple (including juice). Mix the thawed non-dairy topping in a separate wide bowl with the butterscotch dessert topping until uniformly spread. In the non-dairy topping combination, stir the apple/pineapple mixture. Add butterscotch chips and unsalted peanuts. Stir and serve.

## 382- Sweet Mascarpone and Berries

Preparation time: 20 minutes

Cooking Time: 0 minutes

Servings: 6

Difficulty Level: Medium

## Nutritional Information:

Calories: 735 kcal, protein: 11 g, carbohydrates: 24 g, Fat: 6 g, Cholesterol: 0 mg, Fiber: 5 g, Sodium: 81 mg, Potassium: 118 mg, Phosphorus: 18 mg, Calcium: 20 mg

## Ingredients:

- 1/2 cup + 2 tsp of sugar
- 2 cups of mascarpone cheese
- 1 tbsp lemon or orange zest
- 1/4 cup of balsamic vinegar
- 1-pint strawberries

## Instructions:

Combine citrus zest, cheese, and 1/2 cup sugar until combined and smooth. Mix balsamic vinegar, sugar, and berries, and for 10 minutes, marinade it. Add these berries into dessert dishes and cover each with more berries and mascarpone.

## 383- Strawberry Pie

Preparation time: 10 minutes

Cooking Time: 20 minutes

Servings: 8

Difficulty Level: Medium

## Nutritional Information:

Calories: 212 kcal, protein: 1 g, carbohydrates: 40 g, Fat: 5.4 g, Cholesterol: 15 mg, Fiber: 2 g, Sodium: 104 mg, Potassium: 141 mg, Phosphorus: 24 mg, Calcium: 20 mg

## Ingredients:

- 4 cups of strawberries,
- One pie shell, 9" size: unbaked
- 3 tbsp of cornstarch
- 1 cup of sugar
- 8 tbsp of whipped topping (optional)
- 2 tbsp of lemon juice

## Instructions:

Bake the pie shell as instructed on the packet. Set to cool aside. Mash 2 cups of strawberries and add butter, lemon juice, and cornstarch to the mixture. Layer the ingredients in a medium casserole dish. Cook over medium heat until the mixture is thick and clear; keep stirring. Let it cool. Cut and add the leftover strawberries to the cooled mixture. Pour into the cooled pie shell. Cover it and put it in the refrigerator. If required, serve with whipped topping.

## 384- Lemon-Raspberry Sauce

Preparation time: 10 minutes

Cooking Time: 0 minutes

Servings: 8

Difficulty Level: Easy

## Nutritional Information:

Calories: 27 kcal, protein: 0 g, carbohydrates: 7 g, Fat: 3 g, Cholesterol: 0 mg, Fiber: 7 g, Sodium: 0 mg, Potassium: 2 mg, Phosphorus: 0 mg, Calcium: 6 mg

## Ingredients:

- 1/4 cup of sugar
- 6 ounces frozen raspberries; partially thawed.
- 2 tbsp of water
- 1 tbsp of lemon juice

## Instructions:

Blend all the ingredients until smooth and thicker. You can also use other berries, such as blackberries, strawberries, or blueberries. For the perfect sweetness, adjust the sugar.

## 385- Microwave Berry Jam

Preparation time: 5 minutes

Cooking Time: 5-10 minutes

Servings: 16

Difficulty Level: Easy

## Nutritional Information:

Calories: 41 kcal, protein: 0 g, carbohydrates: 10 g, Fat: 0 g, Cholesterol: 0 mg, Fiber: 0 g, Sodium: 0 mg, Potassium: 24 mg, Phosphorus: 3 mg, Calcium: 3 mg

## Ingredients:

- 3/4 cup of granulated sugar
- 1 cup of mashed berries (any kind or combination)
- 1 tsp of lemon juice
- 1/4 tsp of unsalted butter

## Instructions:

Place the ingredients and combine them in a microwave-proof dish. Microwave on high for 5 minutes (for strawberry:4 minutes). Stir it and microwave for 5 more minutes (4 for Strawberries). Place in a lid or plastic wrap cover jar and refrigerate it.

## 386- Orange and Cinnamon Biscotti

Preparation time: 10 minutes

Cooking Time: 50 minutes

Servings: 18 cookies

Difficulty Level: Medium

## Nutritional Information:

Calories: 149 kcal, protein: 2 g, carbohydrates: 22 g, Fat: 6 g, Cholesterol: 34 mg, Fiber: 0.5 g, Sodium: 76 mg, Potassium: 53 mg, Phosphorus: 28 mg, Calcium: 9 mg

## Ingredients:

- ½ cup of unsalted butter
- 1 cup of sugar
- 2 tsp of orange peel: grated.
- 1 tsp of vanilla extract
- 2 large eggs
- 1 tsp of cream of tartar
- 2 cups of all-purpose flour
- 1 tsp of ground cinnamon
- ¼ tsp of salt
- ½ tsp of baking soda

## Instructions:

Spray 2 baking sheets with non-stick cooking spray. In a wide cup, beat the sugar and unsalted butter until well combined. At a time, add one egg, and beat them well. Whisk together the orange peel and vanilla. Combine the flour, tartar cream, baking soda, cinnamon, and salt in a medium-size dish. To the butter mixture, add the dry ingredients and combine until blended.

Slice the dough into two halves. Place each half on a sheet that has been prepared. Shape each half into a log 3 inches wide with lightly floured hands. Bake for 35 minutes until the dough logs are firm to the touch. Take the dough logs from the oven and cool them for 10 minutes. Shift logs to work surface. Use a serrated knife to split it into 1/2-inch-thick slices diagonally. On baking sheets, place cut side down.

Bake for about 12 minutes until the bottoms are golden. Flip over the biscotti; bake for 12 minutes until the bottoms are golden. Before serving, place it on a wire rack and cool it.

## 387- Strawberry Cheesecake

Preparation time: 10 minutes

Cooking Time: 60 minutes

Servings: 8

Difficulty Level: Medium

### Nutritional Information:

Calories: 493 kcal, protein: 8 g, carbohydrates: 35 g, Fat: 10 g, Cholesterol: 5 mg, Fiber: 4 g, Sodium: 468 mg, Potassium: 159 mg, Phosphorus: 164 mg, Calcium: 20 mg

### Ingredients:

- 1 stick of unsalted butter, melted.
- Two packs of crushed graham crackers.
- 1/2 cup of sugar
- 16 oz cream cheese softened.
- 1 tbsp of vanilla extract
- 4 eggs

### Instructions:

Preheat the oven to 325°F. Mix the butter and graham crackers until completely combined.

Spread the mixture in the desired pan evenly (cake pan, pie pan, or springform pan).

Whisk the cream cheese, vanilla, sugar, and eggs until thoroughly mixed and pour onto the crust. Bake for 45-60 minutes or once cooked in the middle (no longer jiggles). Let it cool for three hours.

## 388- Lemon Mousse

Preparation time: 30 minutes

Cooking Time: 10 minutes

Servings: 6

Difficulty Level: Medium

### Nutritional Information:

Calories: 258 kcal, protein: 6 g, carbohydrates: 28 g, Fat: 14 g, Cholesterol: 158 mg, Fiber: <1 g, Sodium: 52 mg, Potassium: 91 mg, Phosphorus: 77 mg, Calcium: 38 mg

### Ingredients:

- ¾ cup of sugar
- 4 large eggs
- 1¼ ounce of gelatin: unflavored
- ¾ cup of heavy cream
- ¼ cup of water
- 1 tbsp of lemon zest (from 2 lemons)
- ½ cup of lemon juice

### Instructions:

Separate egg yolks and place them in separate bowls from the egg whites. Add half of the sugar to a big mixing bowl, and egg yolks are added to the sugar. Beat it at high speed for 5 minutes using an electric mixer.

In a small saucepan, add water and place it over low heat. Add the gelatin and stir until it is dissolved continuously. Remove from the heat and leave for 2 minutes to cool.

Beat the lemon juice and zest with the electric mixer into the whipped egg yolks until well mixed. Mix the dissolved gelatin into the egg yolk mixture through a wooden spoon. Mix and chill for 10 minutes (until the mixture coats the back of the spoon).

Beat the egg whites with the electric mixer at high speed in a stainless or glass bowl and add the remaining sugar (2 tablespoons) at a time. Beat for around 3 to 5 minutes until the whites are firm.

Fold the whipped whites into the dense yolk mixture with a wooden spoon. Beat the cream with the electric mixer in a separate bowl at medium-high speed, until quite thick, for around 5 minutes. Fold in the egg mixture with the whipped cream. Pour into individual bowls for serving and refrigerate for 1 hour. Serve it.

# 389- Honeyed Carrots & Leeks

Preparation time: 5 minutes

Cooking Time: 10 minutes

Servings: 6

Difficulty Level: Easy

## Nutritional Information:

Calories: 108 kcal, protein: 1 g, carbohydrates: 20 g, Fat: 9 g, Cholesterol: 7 mg, Fiber: 4 g, Sodium: 75 mg, Potassium: 256 mg, Phosphorus: 39 mg, Calcium: 7 mg

## Ingredients:

- 1 lb. washed baby carrots,
- 1/2 cup of sliced leeks
- 1 tablespoon of honey
- 1 tsp. of brown sugar: granulated
- 1 lemon, zested.
- 2 Tbsp of lemon juice
- 1 tsp. of olive oil

## Instructions:

Combine the carrots, sugar, leeks, honey, lemon juice, and oil in a pan and cook for 5 minutes over medium heat by covering it with a lid. Uncover and cook until the carrots are tender, about 2 minutes.

# 390- Easy Trifle

Preparation time: 30 minutes

Cooking Time: 20 minutes

Servings: 8

Difficulty Level: Medium

## Nutritional Information:

Calories: 173 kcal, protein: 3.5 g, carbohydrates: 32.9 g, Fat: 0.8 g, Cholesterol: 0 mg, Fiber: 1.4 g, Sodium: 92.1 mg, Potassium: 242.1 mg, Phosphorus: 175 mg, Calcium: 40 mg

## Ingredients:

- 1 sachet custard powder; 75g/3oz
- One Swiss sponge roll: small plain
- 3 tbsp of sherry (optional)
- 1 can of mandarins' pieces in juice: drained; 400g/16oz
- 4 squares of grated chocolate,
- 1/4-pint/150ml double cream

## Instructions:

Pour sachet into measuring jar to make the custard and add the boiling water to the 300 ml or 1/4-pint mark. Stir until creamy and smooth with a fork and leave to set. Slice the Swiss roll into pieces and use 1 wide or 4 individual serving platters to cover the base. Sprinkle the sherry over the Swiss roll, if used. Spread 6 segments of the mandarin equally over the Swiss roll. Over the fruit, pour the custard. The double cream is whipped and poured over the custard. Garnish with some grated chocolate and a little reserved mandarin.

## 391- Glazed Carrots

Preparation time: 10 minutes

Cooking Time: 20 minutes

Servings: 4

Difficulty Level: Easy

### Nutritional Information:

Calories: 97 kcal, protein: 1 g, carbohydrates: 12 g, Fat: 5 g, Cholesterol: 11 mg, Fiber: 1.8 g, Sodium: 150 mg, Potassium: 214 mg, Phosphorus: 24 mg, Calcium: 23 mg

### Ingredients:

- 1 tbsp of sugar
- 2 carrots: medium
- 1 tsp of cornstarch
- 1/4 tsp of ground ginger
- 1/8 tsp of salt
- 2 tbsp of butter
- 1/4 cup of apple juice

### Instructions:

Cut the carrots into strips that are 1 inch wide. Put the carrots and 1/4 of a cup of water in a jar. Until slightly tender, cover and cook. Place the salt, sugar, ginger, cornstarch, melted butter, and apple juice together. Pour the pasta and water over the carrots. Cook for 10 minutes, stirring regularly, or until the mixture thickens.

## 392- Baked Apples

Preparation time: 10 minutes

Cooking Time: 30 minutes

Servings: 2

Difficulty Level: Easy

### Nutritional Information:

Calories: 312 kcal, protein: <1 g, carbohydrates: 53 g, Fat: 13 g, Cholesterol: 31 mg, Fiber: 5 g, Sodium: 16 mg, Potassium: 249 mg, Phosphorus: 32 mg, Calcium: 47 mg

### Ingredients:

- 1 tbsp of lemon juice
- 4 apples
- 1 tsp of vanilla essence
- 4 chopped finely dried dates,
- 12 chopped almonds finely,
- ½ tsp of cinnamon or mixed spice
- 2 tbsp of brown sugar

### Instructions:

Preheat the oven to 180 degrees Fahrenheit. Remove the core from the center and assemble it in a baking dish(ceramic), keeping the apples intact. Drizzle the middle of each apple with lemon juice. Combine the vanilla essence, brown sugar, dates, spices, and almonds. Place the mixture into the center of each apple. Cover the dish with foil and cook for fifteen minutes. Remove the foil and cook for 15 more minutes or until the apples are tender. Use 2 teaspoons of custard to eat with each apple.

## 393- Quick Stem Ginger Ice Cream

Preparation time: 30 minutes

Cooking Time: 0 minutes

Servings: 7

Difficulty Level: Medium

### Nutritional Information:

Calories: 303 kcal, protein: 3.50 g, carbohydrates: 30.3 g, Fat: 18.30 g, Cholesterol: 64 mg, Fiber: 1.4 g, Sodium: 45 mg, Potassium: 100 mg, Phosphorus: 75 mg, Calcium: 150 mg

## Ingredients:

- 70g stem ginger: chopped.
- 500ml double cream
- 4 spoons of stem ginger syrup
- ½ fresh scraped vanilla pod.

## Instructions:

In an electric mixer jar or a wide bowl, pour the double cream and whisk until firm peaks begin to form. Add the minced ginger, squashed vanilla pod, and syrup. Mix well and put in an appropriate bowl that will fit in the freezer. Take out the ice cream after around 20 minutes and swirl it. Leave for roughly 1 hour, then serve.

# 394 Spiced Pears

Preparation time: 1 hour 10 minutes

Cooking Time: 20 minutes

Servings: 12

Difficulty Level: Easy

## Nutritional Information:

Calories: 85 kcal, protein: 0 g, carbohydrates: 19 g, Fat: 1 g, Cholesterol: 0 mg, Fiber: 2.6 g, Sodium: 10 mg, Potassium: 130 mg, Phosphorus: 11 mg, Calcium: 16 mg

## Ingredients:

- 3/4 cup of brown sugar
- 6 pears (medium) peeled and sliced.
- 1-1/2 tsp rum extract
- 2 tbsp crystallized ginger
- 1/4 tsp ground cinnamon
- 1 tbsp margarine
- 1/8 tsp allspice: ground

## Instructions:

Preheat the oven to 350° F. Place pear slices in an 11" x 7" x 2" baking dish. Combine ginger,

brown sugar, rum extract, all spices, and cinnamon. Sprinkle the mixture of brown sugar and margarine pieces over the pears. For 20 minutes, bake. Refrigerate for 1 hour or more to be served chilled or serve hot.

# 395- Baked French Toast Custard

Preparation time: 10 minutes

Cooking Time: 50 minutes

Servings: 4

Difficulty Level: Medium

## Nutritional Information:

Calories: 450 kcal, protein: 16 g, carbohydrates: 65 g, Fat: 14 g, Cholesterol: 0 mg, Fiber: 0.8 g, Sodium: 390 mg, Potassium: 221 mg, Phosphorus: 111 mg, Calcium: 80 mg

## Ingredients:

- 1/2 cup of sugar
- Four slices of Italian bread. sliced 1/2" thick
- powdered sugar or sweetener: non-calorie, optional
- 2 cups of liquid egg substitute: low cholesterol
- 4 cups of rice milk, non-enriched
- 1 teaspoon of almond extract
- 4 tablespoons of margarine: unsalted, melted.
- 1 teaspoon of cinnamon

## Instructions:

Coat the bottom and sides of a 9" x 13" baking tray with margarine or non-stick cooking spray. Arrange the bread slices on a sheet at the bottom of the plate. Mix non-enriched rice milk, melted margarine, egg substitute, sugar, cinnamon, and almond extract in a bowl, and sprinkle over bread slices. Use plastic wrap to protect the pan and refrigerate overnight. Preheat the oven to 350° F.

Put the pan in the oven and bake for 40 to 50 minutes until the knife comes out clean when inserted in the middle. Serve it warm. If needed, sprinkle with powdered sugar or non-caloric sweetener.

# 396- Butter Muffins

Preparation time:10 minutes

Cooking Time: 25 minutes

Servings: 6

Difficulty Level: Easy

## Nutritional Information:

Calories: 438 kcal, protein: 7.3 g, carbohydrates: 56 g, Fat: 18 g, Cholesterol: 104 mg, Fiber: 1.2 g, Sodium: 516 mg, Potassium: 107 mg, Phosphorus: 65 mg, Calcium: 40 mg

## Ingredients:

- 1 (8-oz.) container of sour cream
- 1 cup of butter or margarine: unsalted, melted.
- 2 cups of self-rising flour

## Instructions:

Stir all ingredients together before blending. Pour batter into a miniature muffin pan that is lightly greased. Bake for 25 minutes at 350 ° or until lightly browned.

# 397- Blueberry Baked Bread

Preparation time: 10 minutes

Cooking Time: 20 minutes

Servings: 6

Difficulty Level: Medium

## Nutritional Information:

Calories: 373 kcal, protein: 11 g, carbohydrates: 69 g, Fat: 4 g, Cholesterol: 73 mg, Fiber: 3 g, Sodium: 399 mg, Potassium: 176 mg, Phosphorus: 142 mg, Calcium: 33 mg

## Ingredients:

- ¼ cup of water (for frozen berries)
- 1-quart blueberries,
- 1 tsp of lemon juice
- 1 pinch nutmeg
- ½ cup of sugar
- 1 pinch cinnamon
- 3 slices of bread are buttered and spread with sugar and cinnamon on both sides.
- 1 tbsp margarine

## Instructions:

Heat the oven to 425°F. Under cold running spray, wash the blueberries. Add all ingredients except bread to a saucepan. Just get it to a simmer. In a shallow baking tray, pour the blueberry mixture; cover with bread sliced. Bake until golden brown (10 minutes).

# 398- Litchi Sorbet

Preparation time:5minutes(8 hours; freezing time)

Cooking Time: 0 minutes

Servings:4

Difficulty Level: Easy

## Nutritional Information:

Calories: 95 kcal, protein: 2 g, carbohydrates:23 g, Fat:0g, Cholesterol: 0 mg, Fiber: 1 g, Sodium: 15 mg, Potassium: 207mg, Phosphorus: 36mg, Calcium: 5 mg

## Ingredients

- 2 tbsp of powdered sugar

- 1 lb. fresh litchis; peeled & pitted or 14 oz canned litchis
- 1 pasteurized egg white
- For Garnish: lemon wedge, thinly sliced

## Instructions:

Put litchi flesh and sugar in a blender or food processor and process to a puree. Press the puree through a fine strainer to remove any remaining solids. Transfer to a freezer-proof container and freeze for 3 hours. Turn the mixture into the blender or processor and process until slushy. With the motor running, add the egg white. Return mixture to a freezer-proof container and freeze for 8 hours/overnight. Puree sorbet in blender right before serving, garnish with thinly sliced lemon.

## 399- Brie and Cranberry Chutney

Preparation time: 10 minutes

Cooking Time: 15-20 minutes

Servings: 10

Difficulty Level: Medium

## Nutritional Information:

Calories: 204 kcal, protein: 6 g, carbohydrates: 27 g, Fat: 8 g, Cholesterol: 28 mg, Fiber: 1.9 g, Sodium: 184 mg, Potassium: 118 mg, Phosphorus: 65 mg, Calcium: 74 mg

## Ingredients:

- 1/3 cup of water
- Fresh cranberries: 12 ounces
- 1/2 cup of brown sugar
- 1 tsp of dry mustard
- 1/2 cup of sugar
- 1 tsp of cinnamon
- 1 tsp of cloves
- 30 crackers: low sodium
- 1 tsp of nutmeg
- Brie cheese: 8 ounces

- 1 tsp allspices

## Instructions:

Preheat the furnace to 350° F. Wash the fresh cranberries and drain them. Heat the water in a large skillet for 5 minutes and add the fresh cranberries. Heat until the cranberries begin to burst. Add brown and white sugar (or Splenda). Add the seasoning and gently mix. Remove from the heat. Allow the chutney to cool. Remove Brie's wheel from the wrapper. Cut out a circle and lift out the rind from the middle to expose the Brie inside, keeping a half-inch boundary of the rind on top of the wheel. Put Brie on a baking sheet and place it in the oven until the cheese is partially melted and the surface is sticky. Take Brie out of the oven and put it on a plate. Pour hot chutney on Brie and enjoy with a choice of crackers low in sodium.

## 400- Chocolate Zucchini Cake

Preparation time: 10 minutes

Cooking Time: 50 minutes

Servings: 24 slices

Difficulty Level: Easy

## Nutritional Information:

Calories: 158 kcal, protein: 2.5 g, carbohydrates: 24 g, Fat: 6.5 g, Cholesterol: 0 mg, Fiber: 1 g, Sodium: 115 mg, Potassium: 109 mg, Phosphorus: 45 mg, Calcium: 20 mg

## Ingredients

- ½ cup margarine
- 1 ¾ cup sugar
- 2 eggs
- 1 tsp vanilla
- ½ cup and 2 tbsp milk
- 1 tbsp lemon juice
- 1 ½ cup white flour
- 1 tsp baking soda

- 4 tbsp cocoa
- ½ tsp salt
- 4 cups zucchini, grated fresh or frozen
- ½ cup walnuts, chopped

## Instructions

Cream sugar and margarine; add vanilla and eggs. Mix it well. Mix milk and lemon juice in a separate bowl and sit for a few minutes. Mix all dry ingredients: cocoa, baking soda, flour, and salt. Fold the flour mixture & milk mixture into the creamed mixture alternatively. Add zucchini and stir it well. Pour it into a greased pan of 9" x 13" (23 cm x 33 cm). Top with walnuts when out of the oven. Bake at 350°F (180°C) for 50 minutes or until the toothpick comes out clean. Best served thoroughly cold.

# Conclusion

The renal diet is supposed to help those who want to live kidney-healthy lifestyle. When renal function is reduced, diet is crucial. The proper diet regulates the metabolism. One may boost the efficacy of the therapy by reducing the level of waste products in the blood. This diet offers the body essential nutrition and energy while working to avoid renal discomfort. The renal diet is based on several fundamental principles. The basic one includes a healthy diet rich in whole grains, fiber, carbs, omega-3 fatty acids, vitamins, and fluids. In this diet, protein should be present but not excessively since the body may convert too much protein into nitrates and carbs. Protein is necessary for tissue repair. Additionally, since the body doesn't need nitrates, the kidneys may eliminate them.

Salt intake must be maintained to a minimum, and blood electrolyte levels should be regularly checked and then properly adjusted. Carbohydrates are essential for energy production and must be consumed correctly. But you need to quit using refined ones and use as many unrefined forms of carbs and whole grains as possible. Note that table salt should only be used in cooking and that too much salt might cause renal hypertension and retention. So, avoid salty meals like sausages, chips, and canned goods. Avoiding colored drinks like colas and foods rich in potassium like bananas, citrus fruits, apricots, and dark leafy green vegetables is important for managing the quantity of phosphorus, especially if blood levels rise. Trans fats and hydrolyzed fats must not be consumed in combination with essential omega-3 fatty acids in your diet. Let your doctor know before starting the diet. As early as the first indications of malnutrition appear, dietary guidance becomes important and should be included in patient monitoring.

In addition to assisting patients in taking responsibility for their diet by helping them set goals, advice should consider personal aspects (family, social environment, psychological concerns).

Made in the USA
Las Vegas, NV
05 March 2023